MANAGEMENT BY OBJECTIVES FOR HOSPITALS

Second Edition

Arthur X. Deegan II
Art Deegan and Associates
Clearwater, Florida

Thomas R. O'Donovan
American Academy of
Medical Administrators
Southfield, Michigan

AN ASPEN PUBLICATION®
Aspen Systems Corporation
Rockville, Maryland
London
1982

Library of Congress Cataloging in Publication Data

Deegan, Arthur X.
Management by objectives for hospitals.

Bibliography: p. 331
Includes index.
1. Hospitals—Administration. 2. Management by objectives. I. O'Donovan, Thomas R. II. Title.
RA971.D43 1982 362.1'1'068 82-3929
ISBN: 0-89443-658-9 AACR2

Publisher: John Marozsan
Editorial Director: Michael Brown
Managing Editor: Margot Raphael
Editorial Services: Jane Coyle
Printing and Manufacturing: Debbie Swarr

Library of Congress Catalog Card Number: 82-3929
ISBN: 0-89443-658-9

Printed in the United States of America

1 2 3 4 5

With love and appreciation
to our wives,
Patricia and Gayle

Table of Contents

Preface .... **xi**

PART I—THE THEORY OF MBO **1**

Chapter 1—MBO: What Is It? **3**

- Two Pillars 3
- The Professional Manager 6
- First Definition of MBO 9
- Total System of Management 16
- Advantages of MBO 20
- Summary 24

Chapter 2—Are You Ready for MBO? **27**

- Obtaining a Self-Profile 28
- Summary 36

Chapter 3—Installation of a Total System in the Hospital **39**

- The Decision to Install 39
- Top Management Training 41
- Training for Department Heads 56
- Training for Other Supervisors 59
- Monthly Report 60
- Evaluation 63
- Summary 64

PART II—THE STRATEGIC PLANNING PART OF MBO 67

Chapter 4—Growing Importance of Planning in Hospitals 69

Background: Historical Perspective 69
Forces Shaping Planning 73
Where Are We Now? 83
Organizing the Planning Function 85
Summary 86

Chapter 5—How to Prepare a Long-Range Master Plan 89

Mission Statement 89
The Organization of the Written Plan for
Your Hospital 95
Summary 114
Appendix 5-A 116
Appendix 5-B 123

PART III—THE OPERATIONAL PLANNING PART OF MBO 135

Chapter 6—How to Set Overall Hospital Annual Objectives 137

Completeness of the Draft 139
Prioritizing the Draft 146
Summary 147

Chapter 7—How to Set Objectives with Individual Managers 149

Basic Assumptions 149
Operational Definition of MBO 150
How to Get Started 157
Summary 162

Chapter 8—How to Identify Key Result Areas 165

What Is a Key Result Area? 165
How to Find KRAs 166
Shared Responsibilities 173
The Role of Staff Persons 174
Summary 175

Chapter 9—How to Write Objectives **177**

The Simplest (Simplistic) Approach 177
Criteria Approach 179
Satisfactory Conditions Approach 180
A Reminder about Styles of Supervision 181
Categories of Objectives 182
Sequence for Consideration of Objectives 188
Summary 190

Chapter 10—How to State Routine Objectives **193**

Format for Routine Objectives 193
Indicators of Success 195
Present Level 201
Desired Results for Next Period 203
The New Boss Exercise 205
Critical Analysis Exercise 210
Summary 214

Chapter 11—How to State Problem-Solving Objectives **215**

Step 1: Identifying the Problem Area 216
Step 2: Determining the Present Level 217
Step 3: Defining a Reasonable Desired Level 218
Step 4: Isolating the Difference 218
Step 5: Brainstorming Possible Causes 220
Step 6: Selecting the Most Crucial Causes 221
Step 7: Developing Alternative Solutions 221
Step 8: Evaluating the Proposed Solutions 222
Step 9: Time and Action Plan 224
Sample Using This Nine-Step Model 224
Problem-Solving Assignment 226
Summary 227

Chapter 12—How to State Innovative Objectives **229**

What Is an Innovative Objective? 229
Format for Innovative Objectives 231
Abandonment 234
Final Examples of the Basic Distinction 235
Summary 238

Chapter 13—How to State Personal Development Objectives 239

Format for Personal Development Objectives 241
Summary 249

Chapter 14—How to Integrate MBO and Quality Assurance 251

Background 251
Comparison: QA and MBO 253
What and Who of a QA Program 254
Implementing a Hospitalwide Quality Assessment Program 258
Summary 262
Appendix 14-A 263
Appendix 14-B 265
Appendix 14-C 269

PART IV—THE BUDGETING AND EVALUATING PARTS OF MBO 273

Chapter 15—How to Budget for Objectives 275

Decision Packages 276
Timing of the Budgetary Process 287
Summary 288

Chapter 16—How to Monitor Progress toward Objectives 289

Reporting Techniques 290
Keeping Current 292
Ways to Follow Up 295
Shot-in-the-Arm Examples 296
Summary 298

Chapter 17—How to Evaluate by Objectives 299

Reasons for Formal Performance Appraisal 299
Step-by-Step Procedure 303
Summary 307

Chapter 18—Implementation Strategies **309**

Summary 321

Chapter 19—How to Evaluate the Success of Your Implementation of MBO **323**

Summary 330

Bibliography **331**

Index **335**

Preface

The introduction to the first edition of this book took a lead from national journals and reports of governmental agencies citing the health care industry for its structure that encourages overuse of resources and discourages price competition. Prevalent conditions included:

- large dollar outlays, which might enhance the apparent quality of health care but have not been statistically proven to be the case
- lack of awareness on the part of the consumer of what health care costs are, since over two-thirds of such payments are made by insurance companies or the government
- physician independence in determining the tests, drugs, length of hospital stay, and the like required for patient care
- the "incentive structure of the industry," which appears to encourage waste because hospitals are typically paid on a "cost reimbursement" basis and thus lack reason to hold down spending
- lack of price competition among health care facilities
- the tendency for hospitals to vie with one another by increasing in size, technological sophistication, or "prestige"

Such accusations die hard; hence, five years later hospital managers are still hearing the same charges. Some wonder why the charges are addressed to them when they themselves feel caught up in these same inefficient structures and seem able to do little about them. We would like to say to them: "To whom else can we look for change?" It was the decisions of hospital managers that helped create the industry as it is; it will be the decisions of hospital managers in handling the awesome responsibilities thrust upon them by this still growing, third largest industry in the country that will create a more effective industry.

This book is intended as an aid to them in accomplishing the transformation needed. Taking the principles of a results-oriented approach to management as first practiced in business and industry, we have attempted to describe and illustrate where possible a total system of management for the hospital chief executive officer (CEO) and department manager. We hope thereby to state the case for management by objectives (MBO) completely in hospital terminology, to use only examples from hospital work.

Since the first edition we have had the opportunity to work firsthand with many more health care facilities in implementing our approach to MBO. We are convinced that while our approach is not the only valid way to manage by objectives, the procedures we outline have been proven to be effective where they are put into practice substantially intact.

At the same time we have found with the help of practicing executives that there are always ways to improve on a system. We have attempted to incorporate many improvements in what we recommend in this second edition. In doing so we again wish to thank the many hospital managers whose ideas and examples have been incorporated in this book. Their number is too great to list individually, but thanks are owed them all for their contributions. In truth, this is their book!

Many readers have gone out of their way to make special mention of the style of writing used in the earlier edition. As opposed to most "texts," we write in dialogue form. We shall be talking *to* you in the second person as though we are present with you in the same room and talking to you, asking you questions, and pausing from time to time to ask you to complete some work assignment or exercise.

We have reorganized the chapters into what we hope will be a more logical sequence to get across the idea of MBO as a total system of management and not simply an operational method of controlling day-to-day activities, separate somehow from long-range planning and from the budgeting process. In particular, we would call the following to your attention:

- Part II has been added to highlight the strategic planning part of MBO. It traces the historical development of long-range planning in hospitals and provides detailed help in the preparation of a long-range master plan.
- In Part III almost all the examples have been changed or updated. Chapter 14 is entirely new to show how to integrate a hospitalwide quality assurance program with MBO.

- Almost all of Part IV is entirely new. There is a chapter on integrating the budget with MBO, a chapter on monitoring progress in reaching objectives, and a chapter reporting on an objective way of evaluating the success or failure of implementing your system of MBO.
- The appendixes are also entirely new.

One final word as to why we continue to feel our approach to MBO is worthy of your consideration. One CEO who used this approach for over four years described his satisfaction this way:

> I have always been plagued as President of this organization with two major impediments to progress: ambiguity of expectations and the shortness of the corporate memory. Through negotiation of objectives we no longer have ambiguity as to what is expected. Through adopting this formalized way of recording those negotiated objectives on paper for review purposes we have no longer got to trust our memory.

Part I

The Theory of MBO

Chapter 1

MBO: What Is It?

Several years ago when one of us was teaching at the University of Michigan, a group of British businessmen came to a seminar on management by objectives and said, "This is the twelfth seminar we have attended in your country on this same subject. So far we have received eleven different ideas of what MBO is. Are you going to give us a twelfth?"

Perhaps you have had a similar experience, for it is hardly possible to attend any management conference these days without hearing some reference to MBO. To hear some talk, MBO is primarily an attitude, a state of mind, a philosophy. To hear others, MBO is primarily a matter of filling out forms or meeting deadlines. Still others seem to imply MBO is limited to a new appraisal system, an executive development program, or a modern compensation scheme.[1]

Actually, MBO is all of these. It is a total system of management, an attempt to incorporate all the things a manager ought to be doing into an organized effort. It is not any *one* of the many tools a manager will find helpful from one situation to the next; it is the whole toolbox. This makes it unnecessary to "learn a new method of managing;" no matter what your favorite or most successful management technique, there is probably room for it in MBO.

TWO PILLARS

We would prefer to answer the question "What is MBO?" by describing what it is in those organizations that seem to be most effective with it. Among the successful users of MBO, the system seems to rest squarely on two firm supports or pillars: one theoretical, the other practical (Figure 1-1). Pillar I suggests that there is a solid conceptual foundation for MBO;

Figure 1-1 Two Pillars of MBO

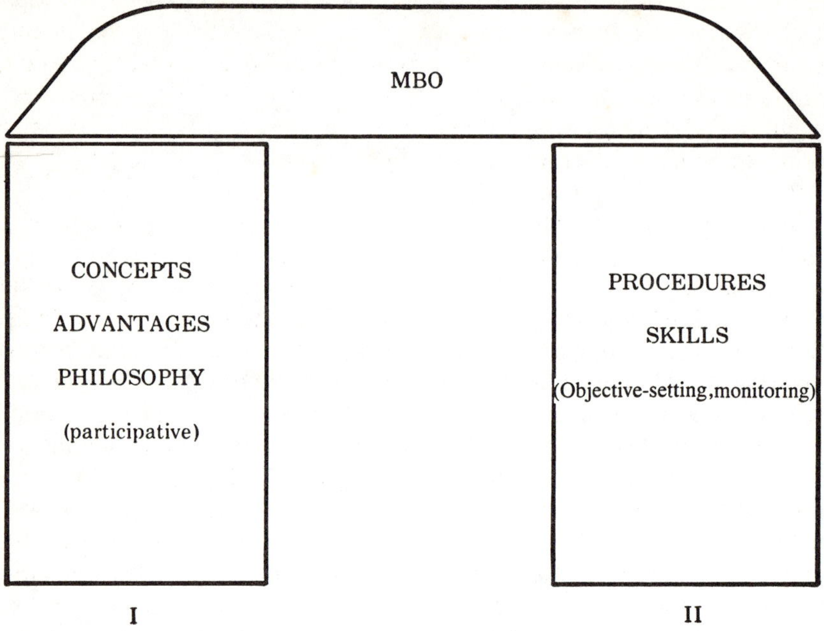

it did not fall out of the clouds fully developed: it emerged from recent findings of students and practitioners of management. It probably would not have the appeal it has today were it not the outgrowth of the work done by certain scholars in the last several decades.

In this sense, MBO owes much to Douglas McGregor and his theory X and Y, to Robert Blake and the managerial grid, to Fred Herzberg's maintenance-motivation factors, and to Rensis Likert and his four systems of management, not to mention Frederick W. Taylor's school of scientific management and Elton Mayo's human relations findings.[2–7]

Further, there are definitely certain advantages to be gained by the users of MBO, benefits for both the individual manager and for the organization. Not to be aware of these advantages, not to keep them in mind as one embarks on a program of implementing MBO, not to set them up as criteria for the subsequent evaluation of the usefulness of MBO would be to risk obtaining minimal results from the system. There are countless managers who have tried MBO and report dissatisfaction with it; often it is because they picked up a tool intended to do one thing and complained it didn't do something else, much like complaining that a thermometer isn't worth very much because it doesn't tell one's blood pressure.

The final part of this theoretic pillar is the particular philosophy that differentiates MBO from other systems of management, what we today call a belief in participative management. Getting into MBO is a deliberate attempt on the part of senior management to involve as many people as possible in the decision-making process, to force decision making down through the organization, to let people have more say about their work as a means of doing a better job in carrying out the mission of the total group. For that reason, the promise of MBO is often like the promise of a new era: great if it works out that way, but totally demoralizing if the promise is not kept. For that reason also, MBO is not necessarily everyone's cup of tea; it is not a panacea for all ills or for all managers. To recognize this clearly at the outset will prevent misconceptions about what it can do and will serve to explain why it is not always successful. For the hospital manager, this will mean that MBO is much like any health care procedure: it works for some, but it is not the only treatment that could be prescribed.

Recognizing ahead of time the particular philosophy that is built into MBO, we are in a better position to tell whether we have the right organizational climate for the system to take root and grow. Likewise, managers will be able to assess the probability of being able to use the system effectively; that is, if they take the time to assess their personal philosophy of management, as we will do in the next chapter.

The first pillar, then, means that it will be worth our time to examine the conceptual framework, the advantages we can gain from use of MBO, and the particular philosophy built into the system if we wish to maximize our use of the recommended practical steps contained in the second pillar.

Pillar II concerns the practical elements of MBO. Just as there are those who might ignore the theoretical side of MBO as a system of management, so there are those who would theorize but never be able to put into practice the ideals of the system. They will benefit from our discussion of the procedures that are recommended to make the system work. There are practical steps, in a logical sequence, that others have found realistic in implanting the system, and it will be our function to share these with you, as well as to warn as much as possible about the pitfalls to be avoided in putting these steps into practice.

Further, it will be our contention that certain skills can be learned to make it possible for MBO to be practiced successfully. This will require two attitudes on the part of the practitioner: first, willingness to expend the effort required to acquire the skills in question, and hence, a measure of self-discipline; and second, resignation to the fact that it will take a little time to develop these skills, and therefore, a great deal of patience.

The particular skills necessary to be effective with MBO deal with *objective-setting* and *monitoring progress* towards these objectives once they are set. In addition, your general skills of communicating, negotiating, obtaining agreement, resolving tension, problem solving, and decision making will also be taxed as you use MBO. But what system of management would not require use of these? Acceptance of managerial responsibility in the hospital, whether as a head nurse, controller, radiologist, executive housekeeper, admitting supervisor, or CEO means facing the task of developing these skills. MBO hopes to organize the task and provide help for developing the skills a little more quickly than by osmosis.

All these are acquired skills; hence, as a hospital manager facing the challenge of learning MBO, you are really only facing the challenge of learning to be as professional in your approach to the handling of people as you want to be in providing patient care.

The balance of this chapter will discuss the first pillar; the remainder of the book will cover procedures, techniques, and skills.

THE PROFESSIONAL MANAGER

It has been said that hospital managers are in about the same position today as physicians were 50 or 60 years ago when they realized it takes more to be a professional practitioner of the art of medicine than a few years apprenticeship as an apothecary. Exposure to someone skillful will not guarantee that some of that person's success will rub off and make the apprentice successful. There is a science to be learned. There are procedures that have proven more or less helpful. There are techniques that are accepted as more or less called for by certain diagnoses. New ideas are constantly being developed, and personal judgment can never be replaced by a laboratory formula. But experience and research still save a lot of guesswork on the part of the neophyte.

Then, too, a training period (internship and residency) under closer supervision of a more seasoned professional provides opportunity for building self-confidence in using professional skills before a person is completely on his/her own. All this is basically to enhance the likelihood of excellent results when professional physicians or paraprofessional ancillaries practice their art.

The same is true for the hospital manager. It takes more than several years experience in a nursing unit or working in an ancillary or auxiliary service department to prepare one to be a manager in any of these areas. Years of seniority have nothing to do with the development of the skills required of a manager. Those years might mean better knowledge of the work going on in the department and might have led to highly developed *working* skills, but the manager is now being called upon to exercise a manager's skills, and that's a whole new ballgame.

Lawrence Peter, in what he called "the Peter Principle," described what happens if we confuse these two sets of skills.[8] Simply stated, his dictum is that in a bureaucratic organization people have a tendency to rise to their level of incompetency. That is, people, who do very well in a job where their skills match the requirements of the position are often "rewarded" by being promoted to a job where the only skills they have no longer fit the position requirements, so they perform incompetently.

Is this not what we often do when we take good dieticians and make them directors of food services, or good staff nurses and make them unit supervisors; or sanitation aides and make them housekeeping managers? Before we promote, we should provide an opportunity for the individual to learn the skills of management, which are quite different than the skills of being a worker.

Consider the definition of a manager as found in most introductory texts on the subject. "A manager is a person who gets things done through other people"; "a manager is a person who gets things done through money, material, and personnel"; "a manager is a person who plans, organizes, implements, and controls"; and so forth. To emphasize the distinct contribution of the manager, envision for a moment someone riding a bicycle. Now suppose one were to ask which of the two wheels of the bicycle is the more important. Some opt for the front wheel, pointing out that the front wheel is the one that provides direction for the bicycle. Others would argue for the rear wheel, since that is the one that provides motion to the vehicle. Still others would find it impossible to choose one over the other, since both by definition are important, if we are to have a *bi*cycle (two wheels).

Perhaps the appropriate answer is to say that the question cannot be answered as posed; before being able to select, one must know "more important for what?" If we're asking which wheel is more important in order to provide direction, the obvious answer is the front wheel because the function of the front wheel is to provide direction. If we're asking which wheel is more important in order to provide movement, the obvious answer is the rear wheel because the function of the rear wheel is to provide thrust. But if we're asking which wheel is more important for the total purpose of the vehicle, then it would seem that relative importance is irrelevant, since the total purpose of the bicycle is a combination of motion and guidance, that is, to get one from point A to point B. All the motion in the world from a rear wheel without the guidance of the front would never accomplish the total purpose of the bicycle; and the most sophisticated control mechanism in the world without a power pack from the rear would likewise never make it possible to achieve the total purpose of the bicycle. So relative importance is irrelevant: what is relevant is this: do we have present simultaneously a method to provide thrust and a method to control that thrust—a rear wheel and a front wheel?

There is an analogy between what happens with the bicycle and what happens in any organization. And this is why the fundamental definition of a manager does not change, regardless of the type of organization being managed; it could be a manufacturing firm, a university, the FBI, the Girl Scouts of America, or a hospital! The same thing happens as on a bicycle: namely, there must be present simultaneously a method of providing energy and a method of controlling that energy if we are going to achieve the purpose of the organization, which is defined as a group of people gathered together for a common end.

To designate who is responsible for providing each of these two distinct functions, we have titles or labels that we apply to people. Those responsible for providing guidance, control, and direction like the front wheel of a bicycle are called managers, officers, supervisors, administrators, chiefs, leaders, or some such word, which says nothing about the individuals' importance, but simply defines their function as being one of providing direction. Conversely, those who provide the hustle and bustle, like the rear wheel of a bicycle, are called workers, nonsupervisors, staff, followers, or some such word, which again is not pejorative in any way, for the word chosen simply says that the role of these individuals is to provide the energy under the guidance of others.

The lesson here ought to be obvious: just as a bicycle with only one wheel functioning will never accomplish its purpose, so an organization with only one group of people performing its function will never achieve its purpose. Perhaps you've seen such an organization. In some groups, everybody seems to be on the front wheel, so to speak: there seem to be "all chiefs and no Indians," everybody telling everybody else what to do, and no one left to carry out the instructions, no matter how erudite they might be! In others, the reverse is true: those who belong on the front wheel have abdicated their responsibility and are comfortably riding the back wheel, so that everybody is putting in 10-, 12-, 14-, or 18-hour days, but no one is up on the front wheel providing direction to all that energy being spent, or probably being misspent for lack of guidance.

As you move ahead in your career from lower to higher levels of responsibility, you are expected to spend less of your time and effort doing the work of the department or organization. You are to be less of a doer and more of a manager of others who are the doers. You are to focus less attention on *how* things are done, and more on *what* is done. You are to be less concerned with activities and more concerned with results. MBO as a system of management is going to help you focus less on activities and more on results. It is often called results-oriented management for that reason.

In the past, the distinction between activities and results might not have been so necessary. Then, the best workers or doers might have been the best ones to "put in charge" because they usually continued to be working supervisors anyway and carried the department or the whole hospital by the sheer weight of their own ability to *do* 29 different jobs.

Today, with the advent of specialization and the development of so many professional, semiprofessional, and paraprofessional services, not to mention the pace with which all of these are constantly changing or the added demands of having to meet the requirements of so many licensing bodies or regulatory agencies, it is just not possible to *do* all these jobs; therefore, we have managers who get them done by others. But we still have to be sure that the resulting patient care meets our standards of excellence—and we try to. MBO is simply a system to help us do this more systematically, that is, improve the professionalism of our management team and help us stay on top of things. It is for the hospital manager who realizes that the job of managing a hospital or a department within the hospital is not what it used to be. Because we are in a new environment, new approaches are called for.

You may have heard of the episode in a best-selling novel in which three inhabitants on a small island in the middle of the ocean were asked this question: "What would you do if I told you a great typhoon is coming tomorrow and will swallow up this whole island?"[9] The first inhabitant said he would eat, drink, and be merry in the time remaining. The second inhabitant said he would run to his gods and pray for help. But the third inhabitant said he would seek expert advice on how to breathe under water!

MBO is the way to survive the new management challenges.

FIRST DEFINITION OF MBO

One might say that MBO was developed to assist managers in sorting out the difference between what all too often *is* (putting out fires, being nice to people) and what *ought to be* (accomplishment, anticipation, priorities, results) in terms of how their time is used.

Using the systems language in vogue these days, we can see there must be three elements in management, as there are three elements in any system (Figure 1-2).

In any system there are first of all inputs, or things put into the system. For example, in a computer system, the inputs might be the data fed into the computer, the programs that tell the computer what to do, the people

Figure 1-2 Elements in Any System

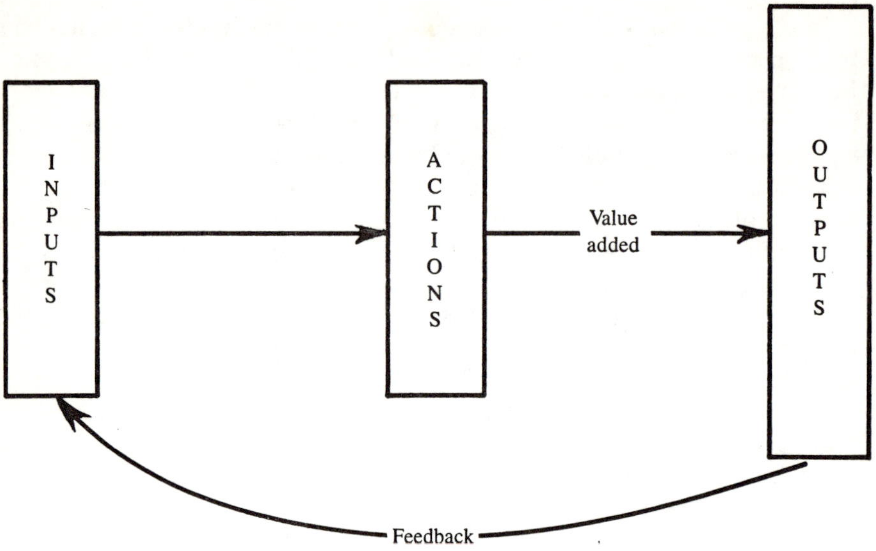

who run the computer, the computer hardware itself, and so forth. The second element is the activity or processing part of the system. In a computer system, to stay with the same example, this refers to the manipulating, rearranging, scoring, printing, and other processes done upon the information fed to the machine. And finally we have outputs, or what comes out the other end of the system. Again, in our computer example, this refers to the printouts, displays, reports, analyses, and the like that the computer provides upon our request.

You will notice in Figure 1-2 that the output box is drawn somewhat larger, suggesting that the intent is to wind up with something that is worth more than the original inputs—"worth," not necessarily in a financial sense, but in terms of whatever values are added to the original inputs by the processing that is done.

Finally, there is a feedback loop in our system, to show that the outputs the first time around are often plowed back into the system as new inputs, or that one person's outputs are often surrendered to another individual as the latter's inputs, and thus the cycle can be repeated over and over again.

Management can be conceived of as such a system with the same three elements and interrelationships. Let us see if we can define the content of each of these three elements in your managerial system for the purpose of noting the essential differences among them. First, you are a manager requiring certain inputs or things put into your hands, in order that you can begin to behave like a manager. See yourself walking around with your hands outstretched, and there's this big funnel in the sky from which certain inputs must come if you are to be able to operate. Let's make a list of some of these.

Question: What are some of the inputs in your management system?
Answer:

You should have answered that your inputs include such things as staff (personnel), money, equipment, facilities of all sorts, buildings, floor space, tools, supplies, time, ideas, information, attitudes, and the like. Some of these are physical, tangible, visible, while others are invisible, intangible, yet very real and very significant. They are all inputs.

Don't use the word *asset* as synonymous with *input*. Sometimes some of those things coming out of the funnel into your hands are not really assets, or at least are not perceived by you as assets; you may see them as liabilities, especially if they somehow curtail your freedom to operate or in any way jeopardize it. For example, rules, policies, laws, and regulations are among your inputs, and you might see them as not very helpful. Or some of the equipment, supplies, buildings (or even people) might not be in the condition you would like them to be, so you consider them a liability. Nonetheless, these are your inputs: they are what you have with which to do your job as a manager. And the wise manager begins by taking stock of the available inputs. Here we just want to be sure not to mislead you in defining the term *input* and the variety of items that belong *by definition* in this box.

Now that you have these inputs to act upon, let's make another list, this time of activities.

Question: What work is done by you and your people using these inputs?
Answer:

You should have answered that your activities include such things as scheduling, budgeting, making patient rounds, distributing medications, giving baths, preparing meals, collecting specimens, paying invoices, purchasing supplies, sweeping floors, planning, motivating, communicating, decision making, problem solving, and the myriad of things you and your people do. You'll notice that we tend to use words ending in *-ing,* the verb form of the word, suggesting that activities mean motion or process. Some of these activities are physical, visible, and tangible, while others are intangible or invisible, but nonetheless very real and very important. You'll also notice that the items in this box can also be divided into positive and negative, as were the inputs. Negative work would be the actions we perform that are counterproductive, that are unsuccessful, that waste some of the resources we began with. This suggests that we may not always be interested in whether an individual works long and hard, but whether that work produces what we desire. The idea may not be to work hard, but to work smart.

This takes us then to the final box in the diagram, the outputs. Let's make a final list.

Question: What are some of the outputs or results of your work activities?
Answer:

You should have listed the products or services you hoped to provide or complete when you engaged in any activity. For example, among the outputs of various hospital work groups would be well patients, clean floors, meals served, charts completed, bills paid, supplies delivered, tests recorded, and so on. Outputs refer to what you made happen, what you accomplished, what you now can point to that did not exist before you began. Some of these results will again be tangible, visible, and physical while others will be less tangible, such as patient satisfaction, the image or reputation of the hospital, staff growth, and so forth. Outputs describe the fruit of your labor in terms of the values you have added to the original resources through the wise selection and implementation of programs of action, through timely and energetic expenditure of energy by you and your people.

These outputs do not always have to be stated in terms of the ultimate results of the organization, the final results for the entire hospital, like patients discharged according to discharge criteria. Outputs may be of an intermediate nature, the results of a given department, or a single individual's results in a short period of time. As a matter of fact, we can take any one of those words ending in *-ing* in the activity box and ask ourselves, "When the activity is over, when the dust has settled so to speak, what have I got to show for it?" The answer will be an output.

The output can also be a negative result, as well as a positive one. That is to say, it could be that the activity did not produce what we wanted it to, or the result might be lower in quality than we desired. Perhaps the patient dies; there might be an employee injured; sometimes people make errors (in distributing medications, in making a diagnosis, in completing a report, in typing a letter, in filling a prescription, and so on). We are not interested yet in whether there is any guilt involved for anything. We are simply defining terms and learning what phenomena go in which of our three boxes in Figure 1-2.

We have described the items in each of the three elements as though they are distinct from one another: certain things are inputs, certain things are activities, and certain things are outputs. This is always by definition, not by our personal choice. These words simply refer to different phenomena in the real world. An input is not an activity, and neither of these is an output. To confuse one with another, to call one by the name of the other is at best a mistake, and at worst harmful to communications. The first two are means to the achievement of the end results, and means are always different from the end they produce. This being the case, we are now ready for the jackpot question. What we have been doing here so far is trying to define MBO. We found that the first word, management, refers to the responsibilities of those who are to ride the front wheel of the bicycle. Now the third word, objectives.

Question: Whenever we hear, see, use the word *objectives,* which box are we discussing?

Answer:

You should have answered, "The output box." *Objectives describe the results we intend to accomplish, what we will have to show for the expenditure of our resources and our energy. When they are still to come, we call them objectives (intended results); when they have already taken place, we call them outputs (actual results).*

This is why we prefer to call the system "management by objectives," whereas others call it "management by goals" or "management by results'' (not to mention ''planning, programming, budgeting system'' or ''planning, evaluation and review,'' etc.). We prefer objectives, because the *o* in objectives reminds us of the *o* in outputs. We are thereby reminded to stay out of what some call the ''input trap'' or ''activity trap,'' calling something an objective when it really is an input or an activity.

For example, some hospital supervisors, when asked for a list of objectives, have been known to state things like the following:

- My objective is another RN for my unit by June 15.
- My objective is another adding machine for the business office by October 30.
- My objective is an additional $50,000 in my budget for next year.
- My objective is another 5,000 square feet of filing space for my department by February 15.
- My objective is acquisition of the Central Supply area by May 1st.

Question: But, what are these: more people, more equipment, more money, more floor space, more authority?

Answer:

You should have said, ''These are inputs.'' People thought they were valid objectives because they put a date on them. But by definition they refer to desired resources. They are a shopping list. They may describe assets you legitimately wish to acquire in order to do your management job well. But they do not in any way describe results, so they are inappropriately called objectives. The trap or danger in continuing to refer to them as objectives comes from what people do when an objective has been identified. That is to say, they marshall all their energies to achieve the identified objectives, for objectives are to be achieved; the attainment of them is a measure of success. We do not wish to encourage people to measure their success simply by the acquisition of resources, without looking ahead to the results achieved by wise use of these resources. To do otherwise is to foster empire building; this is what bureaucracies are made of.

The only time these items might be considered valid objectives is when the nature of the entire job is to acquire them. For example, the purchasing department's job is to purchase supplies, so additional supplies or equipment, to be surrendered to someone else to use, is a valid objective; the personnel department's job is to hire personnel, so another employee, to be given to another manager as an asset, is a valid objective.

Again, other supervisors, when asked for a list of objectives, give answers such as the following:

- My objective is developing a new personnel handbook by next year.
- My objective is conducting an orientation session for all new employees once a month.
- My objective is having a staff meeting with my people once a week.
- My objective is visiting four other hospitals and asking questions about their preadmission procedure.
- My objective is introducing primary care nursing by January 1.
- My objective is to automate patient billing by July 1.

Question: But, what are these: developing handbooks, conducting sessions, having meetings, visiting hospitals, automating procedures?

Answer:

You should have said, "They are activities." They describe what you will be doing; they are a schedule of events; they tell us how busy you are; they are a litany of all the programs you occupy yourself with. At best, they are a list of projects you find important, but in no way should completion of projects, without stating satisfactory conditions for the successful accomplishment of those projects, be accepted as a statement of objectives. The real objectives are the results by way of improvement to be brought about by means of these programs. The means is not to be confused with the end.

Question: Therefore, what are some synonyms for the word *objectives* in the phrase *management by objectives?*

Answer:

You could have used any of these: goals, targets, results, outputs, improvements, benefits, standards of performance, products, criteria of acceptance, but definitely *not* inputs or activities. Our own preference, as mentioned above, is the word *objectives*. And even though we have used goals and objectives rather interchangeably to this point, we shall adopt the word *objective* from now on, thus avoiding needless confusion.

(Some have tried to posit a time difference between goals and objectives, making one a long-range result and the other a short-range result. If this is found to be useful, who can argue with it? The danger might be that not everyone in the organization has a copy of your lexicon, and without an agreement on the meaning of words, there might be a communications problem. Just be sure that what you call a short-run or intermediate result is a real result and not simply a first action step such as hiring people, getting equipment, training staff, etc. These are short-run activities and not results of any time duration.)

Our first definition of MBO then becomes:

> MBO is a system of personal responsibility in which outputs (results) are the only claim on the resources of the organization and outputs (results) are the justification for approving, modifying, or abandoning programs of action.

We will return to the "personal responsibility" part of this definition. For now, we are seeking to keep the relationship among the three elements of the system in the proper order. We are not ignoring inputs or activities. You certainly need resources to do your work, and you certainly should select wisely the programs of action to occupy your time. But it is the results you do or do not accomplish that measure how well you use the assets with which you are entrusted.

TOTAL SYSTEM OF MANAGEMENT

If MBO is to help fulfill management responsibilities in a more professional way, it must be viewed as a total system of management. It ought not to be approached as "one more job I've got to do." Essentially, it is not an addition to your manager's job, but a way of doing what you ought to be doing.

The business firms and other organizations that have been using MBO for some time are quick to point out that minimum results usually come about when managers get the impression that objective-setting is similar to preparing a dollar budget or completing a typical performance appraisal form. That is, if the task of defining objectives is viewed as responding to the request of some staff office (just as the budget is made out "for the controller" and the performance review is completed "for the personnel office"), then it becomes an imposition, an intrusion on the routine of the manager's job, something to be done for someone else's benefit. Obviously this misses the whole point. Even more than a budget or a performance review, the objectives set are for a manager's own use primarily.

How is MBO a way of doing the manager's job? Essentially, it is not a task of putting objectives down on paper; that is only the beginning. As a matter of fact, to get maximum benefits from the system a manager must appreciate the overriding importance of objectives for carrying out *all* his functions of management.

Consider the traditional functions of management as commonly listed in most books on the subject: planning, organizing, directing (coordinating), motivating (actuating), and controlling. To the degree that you can learn a system that will help you identify meaningful, measurable, and communicable objectives, to that degree you will be better able to carry out each of these management functions.

Take *planning*. This is a matter essentially of looking ahead and deciding what results one is going to achieve. Not what one is going to *allow* to happen, but what one is going to try to *make* happen—for there is a decided difference. Ineffective managers simply forecast; they try to predict what the occupancy rate will be, what the length of stay will be, what Blue Cross will allow, what financing terms will be available, and so forth. Effective managers make the same predictions but then ask themselves if these results are what they want to happen. *Then they figure out what they are going to do to change the outcome from what is predicted to what they would prefer it to be.*

Managers who simply look into a crystal ball to do "planning" deserve the annual Christopher Columbus award, because for all intents and purposes they are the same as good old Chris. We are told he set sail from home not knowing where he was going, arrived some place not knowing where he was, and went back home not knowing where he had been! This might be acceptable behavior for an explorer—to set sail and be buffeted this way and that by the winds and waves—but not for a manager.

Managers who wish to set sail for the destination they have in mind will use MBO as a way of clarifying, for everyone's benefit, the occupancy levels, income projections, financing terms, and the like that they realistically would like to achieve; then they will move heaven and earth to get them, realizing they can't control all the variables themselves.

Objectives, then, become the statement of results you intend to achieve. And obviously, the likelihood of achieving results becomes greater when you state specifically what results you seek. By determining meaningful, measurable, and communicable results you are able to plan more effectively.

But MBO doesn't stop there. Take the second function of management, *organizing*. Basically, this refers to putting together the resources a manager has or needs to fulfill responsibilities. It means staffing with the people needed, assigning them proper authority and responsibility, and delegating to them necessary powers to carry out their duties.

How can you evaluate your organizing skill? How will you know the number of people you ought to have as part of your team? How will you know what kind of training to provide for them? How will you know whether you are overstaffed or understaffed? How will you know whether you have delegated enough of your own authority?

The only possible way to answer these questions is through measuring achievement of objectives. You are a good organizer if your organization carries out its work by accomplishing highest priority objectives.

Parenthetically, one might notice how unusual this is. How many managers do you know who put together their organization *after* identifying their objectives? Isn't it more typical when a person is given a management position of higher authority that the boss says: "Here's your new job; and here is your organization: you have this much staff, that much floor space, and these physical facilities. Now, what are you going to do with it?"

If organization flows from objectives, it should be apparent that, to the degree you can learn a system that will help determine meaningful, measurable, and communicable kinds of results, to that degree you will also be assisted in your organizing responsibility.

Take the third managerial function, *directing*. As a manager you probably spend more time fulfilling the directing function than any other one. Why? Because it includes all the day-to-day relationships between you and your people by which you coordinate their activities. It involves the installing, launching, and implementing of the work planned, for which organizational units have been established. It includes operating the programs through systems, procedures, processes, and other means designed for a particular job, whether it's in a nursing unit or supporting department. It involves developing rules, regulations, requirements, and guides for effective operation. It includes the giving of explicit instructions, the preparation of schedules, and the close supervision or inspection of work that is being done. It means supervising the operations to ensure full utilization of personnel, money, materials, facilities, and other resources—with minimum of waste and with concern for high quality at every step of the way.

Once more, we might ask how you will know whether you have done all this well? And, once more it would seem the only logical answer must be, you are directing well if your directions succeed in helping the organization accomplish the objectives considered to be most realistic. Therefore, you are going to be helped in this third managerial function if you learn a system that will develop meaningful, measurable, and communicable objectives because they will then be the guides needed in giving directions.

The fourth management function usually identified is *motivating*. Much has been written about the nature of motivation, but much more still needs to be learned about this most difficult of all management responsibilities. However you choose to define it, motivation must have something to do with understanding what makes people "tick" in any enterprise. It requires an alertness to those basic needs and special interests that, if fulfilled to a considerable extent, lead to job satisfaction. It requires an ability to gauge evidence of dissatisfaction leading to grievances, complaints, absenteeism, poor communication, turnover, and other blocks to providing the quality of service desired.

Solving the motivation riddle means providing management systems, processes, and participation opportunities conducive to good employee morale. It means encouraging in your staff a desire to fulfill their responsibilities as they should. It means understanding incentives and being able to assess their effectiveness and varied success with different types of individuals. It means learning the skills of counseling, appraising, coaching, and training in the development of your subordinates.

One factor common to most motivation research is the connection between individuals' personal objectives and the objectives of their work group. It seems that the way to help people enhance the desire to accomplish the group's goals by performing work well is to show that by doing this they will at the same time accomplish personal objectives. Once again, the system of MBO zeros in on individual motivation because it teaches the personal process for finding the most meaningful, measurable, and communicable kinds of objectives.

The management process is completed through the function of *controlling*. It is commonly agreed that this function really includes two separable components: the act of making a judgment and the determination of any necessary corrective action. If you want your judgment about the work of subordinates to be accepted by them as helpful, you must evaluate them on the basis of acceptable criteria. The best way to evaluate performance is against standards agreed upon *in advance* with them.

Without this means of determining what is "par for the course" you are not in a position to make a meaningful appraisal. *MBO is a process that identifies mutually acceptable standards of performance in advance.*

But with its emphasis on corrective action for the future, MBO goes further. It focuses the attention of both managers and subordinates on how they can constantly seek to improve, rather than simply rehashing past experiences. The point here is that MBO ought not to be seen as primarily a planning tool, or primarily an appraisal tool, or primarily a motivation tool; it is all these and then some. It is an umbrella covering all functions of management—it is a *system* of management.

This view of MBO is essential if the advantages it promises are to be achieved. The literature abounds with illustrations of organizations that began MBO as simply a planning device or simply as a better method of performance appraisal. When that happens, it is almost certain that management will not improve because most people will see it as a threat.

Since we all think we plan, who needs MBO to remind us? One has enough trouble getting most people to accept the concept of evaluation; if MBO is principally a new slant on appraisal, we can expect all kinds of resistance. But MBO is not one more item for the already busy manager; it is a way of doing what is already supposed to be done; it's the whole process of management.

My personal choice is to avoid even the word *program* in connection with MBO. It's not a program because programs come and go; programs occupy a limited amount of our attention and concern. We have safety programs and recruiting programs and cost-cutting programs. These are limited efforts; they are drives for this and that single item of concern, usually in response to a crisis situation. With MBO we are trying to avoid managing by crisis or management by drives or by whim; we are trying to manage by objectives. It is a system, not a program.

Question: Let's summarize: What do we mean when we say MBO is a total system of management?

Answer:

You should have said that MBO ought not to be considered a piece of the manager's job or an addition to it, but that it is intended to be a way of doing the *entire* job. We want to plan by objectives, organize by objectives, direct/supervise people by objectives, motivate by objectives, and evaluate/measure by objectives.

ADVANTAGES OF MBO

As practiced by those who report that they have improved the professionalism of their management team, there are three major advantages of adopting the MBO system: (1) improved planning, (2) improved communications, and (3) improved motivation. If you feel your management team could benefit from improving these three important managerial functions, perhaps MBO can be of help to you. If you are already using MBO (formally or informally), you may want to check out how effectively you are doing so by using these three areas as criteria for judging satisfaction with the system.

Improved Planning

The responsibility of an individual manager to plan was discussed above. But what about the overall planning effort of the entire hospital? Wouldn't it be nice if the plans of the laboratory tied into the plans of the nursing floors? Wouldn't it be nice if the plans of administration tied into your department's goals? Wouldn't it be nice if the plans of each department and section tied into the plans of other departments and sections whose work they affect?

MBO can be a tool to bring about such a *systems* approach to planning. If you use it you will find certain steps and procedures deliberately built into the recommended program that almost force integration of plans up and down in the total hospital and horizontally among the different departments, work groups, and individuals. Do you need to improve planning this way? If so, MBO can help.

Improved Communications

A second major advantage of a smoothly functioning system of MBO is closer communications between several echelons of the management team. Figure 1-3 will be useful to visualize the kind of situation that all too often exists in a hospital, one that can be greatly improved by MBO.

Figure 1-3 Need for Improved Communications

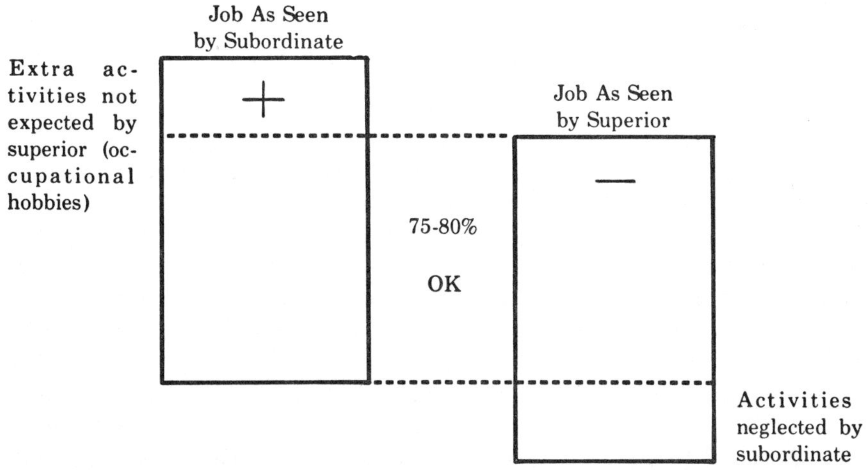

Let department heads or first-line supervisors set down briefly what their major duties are, what the priorities among these duties are, and what the standards are to be used in measuring how well these duties are carried out. Then let their immediate superiors also set down briefly what the subordinates' duties are, what their priorities should be, and what standards are in fact used to evaluate their performance.

Typically, there will be a good deal of agreement about the items on both lists when compared with each other—marked "OK" on Figure 1-3. There will usually also be a certain amount of items that are "extra" (marked "+") on the list of the person doing the work. These are things built into the job to suit one's own talents, perceptions, or understanding of what is expected. Often these are "occupational hobbies" carried over from the last job. On the other hand, there will usually also be a certain number of items that are "lost" (marked "−") from the list of the superior. These are things the subordinate was thought to be doing, things by which the superior intends to measure the subordinate, but which, unfortunately, are not being done.

This communications breakdown between matched pairs of a management team is responsible for many mistakes, oversights, and duplication of effort. We usually run into it when we hear "Oh, I didn't know that's what you wanted." It is often true and always unnecessary.

MBO offers a way to minimize this lack of agreement between levels of management. You will find certain steps and procedures deliberately built into the system to deal with these communications barriers.

Improved Motivation

The third major advantage of MBO is increased motivation for all members of the management team. Of all the responsibilities of a manager, motivating subordinates is usually mentioned as the most important if performance is to be at high standards.

Most managers believe they know a lot about how to motivate their people. That is to say, they *intellectually* know how to motivate: they know that to give a person a pat on the back from time to time is a good way of motivating. They know that giving tangible forms of recognition such as pay increases and promotions is helpful. They realize that increased freedom to make decisions and to monitor one's own performance is also a good way to motivate people.

But knowing this intellectually and putting it into practice can be quite different. Because most managers are busy, because each case is different, and because so many imponderables affect the motivation of subordinates, many managers simply don't get around to putting into practice what they know they ought to do. MBO can help overcome these difficulties. You will find built into the recommended procedures for the practice of MBO certain steps deliberately there because of their motivational impact.

These advantages are from the point of view of the total hospital. Individuals also benefit. Here is how one executive sees them after using MBO for a few years.

MBO benefits the individual supervisor by:

- providing a good coaching framework
- strengthening weak appraisal methodology
- strengthening the supervisor-subordinate relationship
- motivating subordinates

Perhaps the most important benefits accrue to the subordinates:

- Their authorities and responsibilities are clarified.
- They are aware that they will be measured by performance and results rather than personal characteristics.
- They know what is expected of them.
- They experience increased job satisfaction.

At this stage you should also begin to understand that there are several potential pitfalls of the system.

- Employees can become frustrated if they are led to feel that each year increasingly higher goals will be demanded.
- Overemphasis on the achievement of objectives, to the exclusion of more routine and administrative work, can undermine managerial effectiveness; also, employees must not be overwhelmed by what some may call the "sea of paper" in the MBO process.
- The quality of objectives deteriorates at each level if strong coaching and development are not stressed.
- Coaching should not always be left until the time of the annual or quarterly review. If, for example, there is to be an administrative change, coaching should be done at that time.

While we are on the subject of pitfalls, there are other limitations that have been found to exist that should be called to the attention of managers in all industries as they approach MBO.[10,11]

- The system does not appraise and identify potential; therefore, the system places the burden on supervisors to assess lack of results in light of their responsibility for coaching and development.
- The system presumes that workers and their bosses will together establish suitable standards that will serve the company well.
- It implies that bosses understand their limitations and refrain from playing God.
- In action, the system stresses results and does not provide methods of achieving them.

SUMMARY

In this chapter we have attempted to answer the question, "What is MBO?" We have seen that it can be a total system of management and not just a tool for the individual manager. It is as much a way of thinking as it is a set of practical skills.

People generally set objectives for two basic reasons: (1) because the clearer the idea you have of where you are trying to go, the greater the likelihood you will get there; and (2) progress can only be measured in terms of what you are trying to achieve. As an old proverb says, "If you don't know where you're going, any road will get you there." Since most managers find it difficult to be specific about the results they are trying to accomplish, MBO advocates that a system of management that focuses attention on meaningful, measurable, and communicable kinds of results will be of direct benefit to them.[12–14]

Perhaps the best summary of benefits to be derived from the implementation of this system can be found in the quotations of some hospital administrators who have reported their experiences with MBO:

> This program helped us to build close cooperation among all those work groups needed to support one another.

> The program helped me, as administrator, to learn much of what was going on in the various departments about which I had no knowledge before.

> I learned how to replace opinion and casual thought by knowledge, fact, and thorough analysis.

> Now I feel more confident in my ability to assess progress. Some of the hard-to-get-at parts of my job have been reduced to practical units of measurement.

> When we let our people set their own objectives, they surprise us by setting them higher than we would have.
>
> Your approach has helped people in my department see how to achieve their own personal objectives while working toward our institutional objectives.

We must be careful, however, not to overstate our case. MBO is not a cure-all. It will not be effective everywhere. More specifically, it will not help you or your hospital unless both become conditioned for the philosophy built into MBO. What that philosophy is and how organizations and individual managers can determine whether they are ready for MBO will be the subject of the next chapter.

NOTES

1. *Managing by—and with—Objectives* (Chicago: National Industrial Conference Board, Study in Personnel Policy, No. 212, 1968).
2. Douglas M. McGregor, *The Human Side of Enterprise* (New York: McGraw-Hill, 1960).
3. Robert Blake and Jane Mouton, *The Managerial Grid* (Houston: Gulf Publishing Co., 1964).
4. Frederick Herzberg, "One More Time: How Do You Motivate Employees?", *Harvard Business Review,* January–February 1968.
5. Rensis Likert, *New Patterns of Management* (New York: McGraw-Hill, 1961).
6. Frederick W. Taylor, *Scientific Management* (New York: Harper & Bros., 1947).
7. Elton Mayo, *Human Problems of an Industrial Civilization* (New York: Macmillan Co., 1933).
8. Lawrence Peter, *The Peter Principle* (New York: Wm. Marrow & Co., 1969).
9. Leo Rosten, *Captain Newman,* M.D. (New York: Harper & Row, 1961).
10. George S. Odiorne, *Management by Objectives* (New York: Pitman Publishing Co., 1965).
11. Dale D. McConkey, "MBO Works for Managers Who Understand, Apply System," *Hospital Progress,* Sept. 1979.
12. R.D. Arvey, H.D. Dewhirst, and J.C. Boling, "Relationships Between Goal Clarity, Participation in Goal Setting and Personality Characteristics on Job Satisfaction in a Scientific Organization," Appl Psychol 61, no. 1 (1976): pp. 103–5.
13. "The New Industrial Relationships," *Business Week,* May 11, 1981, pp. 84–97.
14. Charles G. Burck, "What Happens When Workers Manage Themselves," *Fortune,* July 27, 1981, pp. 62–69.

Chapter 2

Are You Ready for MBO?

At first glance this question might seem insulting. How can there be a question about the readiness of a manager to use a system of management? Isn't it simply a matter of picking up the tool you feel you want to use and start using it?

Unfortunately, it just doesn't work that easily. There is no panacea to fit every circumstance and every individual. It would be a mistake to approach MBO as though it could be applied immediately in every organization or with every manager.

The previous chapter dealt with the importance of participative decision making as a basic if maximum benefits of MBO are to be realized. But participative management is not everyone's cup of tea. As a matter of fact, tried by the wrong person or in the wrong situation, it can cause havoc.

Shared decision making is a delicate operation requiring controlled conditions for success. It is easily spoiled by contact with authoritarian "germs." Sometimes these bacteria are airborne: they are carried in a person's attitude, not spread by deliberate contamination.

This being the case, the organization and the individual manager will be well advised to ask, "Am I ready for MBO? Is my style of management compatible with the philosophy built into the system? Do we have the management climate necessary to support mutual goal setting? Can I be participative, or have I built up such a history of one-person decision making that it just isn't in me to be otherwise?"

Critics of MBO often cite the gap that exists between the theory as outlined in the preceding chapter and the way too many managers seem to apply the theory. For example,

> Despite the fact that the concept of management by objectives (MBO) has by this time become an integral part of the managerial

> process, the typical MBO effort perpetuates and intensifies hostility, resentment, and distrust between a manager and subordinates. As currently practiced, it is really just industrial engineering with a new name, applied to higher managerial levels, and with the same resistances. Obviously, somewhere between the concept of MBO and its implementation, something has seriously gone wrong. . . .[1]

It is our conviction that malpractice takes nothing away from the values of the system itself. Rather, such instances highlight the necessity for adequate safeguards. Any finely tuned instrument can be abused. The purpose of this chapter is to provide you with a simple means to check your personal preparedness to use the system correctly and to check the management climate in your organization.

OBTAINING A SELF-PROFILE

Exhibit 2-1 is a test of your assumptions regarding people and their work and how to get them to do the work that is expected. You should complete the test by checking the appropriate column for each of the 15 statements before reading the explanation that follows the figure. Two simple ground rules should be followed in completing the test:

1. Read each statement and immediately place a check in one of the four columns. It is your assumptions, your predispositions, your subconscious judgment that are being measured—not your carefully reasoned response. Therefore, answer at once, upon reading, not after making qualifications of the statements or by seeking the "right" answer. In this test, there are no right or wrong answers. There are only *your* answers. The best answer is the one that best describes what you actually believe. Any other answer will serve only to cloud the picture we are looking for—your instinctive pattern of behavior.
2. Try to think of "people" in this test in a rather general sense. Don't think of specific individuals, whether they be "strong right arms" or "constant thorns in your side." We are looking for your general pattern of behavior. The image you project to others is what we seek here. The object of the test is for you to look in a mirror to see yourself as others see you, as you really are in your unguarded moments, not the way you wish you were.

Exhibit 2-1 Test Your Own Assumptions Regarding People and Their Work

(Check one)	*Strongly Disagree*	*Disagree*	*Agree*	*Strongly Agree*
1. Almost everyone could probably improve his/her job performance quite a bit if he/she really wanted to.	______	______	______	______
2. It is unrealistic to expect people to show the same enthusiasm for their work as for their leisure activities.	______	______	______	______
3. Even when given encouragement by the boss, very few people show the desire to improve themselves on the job.	______	______	______	______
4. If you give people enough money, they are less likely to worry about such intangibles as status or recognition.	______	______	______	______
5. Usually when people talk about wanting more responsible jobs, they really mean they want more money and status.	______	______	______	______
6. Because most people don't like to make decisions on their own, it is hard to get them to assume responsibility.	______	______	______	______
7. Being tough with people will usually get them to do what you want.	______	______	______	______
8. A good way to get people to do more work is to crack down on them once in a while.	______	______	______	______
9. It weakens a person's prestige whenever he/she has to admit that a subordinate has been right and he/she has been wrong.	______	______	______	______
10. The most effective supervisor is one who gets the results expected, regardless of the methods he/she uses in handling people.	______	______	______	______

Exhibit 2-1 continued

(Check one)	*Strongly Disagree*	*Disagree*	*Agree*	*Strongly Agree*
11. It is too much to expect that people will try to do a good job without being prodded by their boss.	______	______	______	______
12. The boss who expects his/her people to set their own standards for superior performance will probably find they don't set them very high.	______	______	______	______
13. If people don't use much imagination and ingenuity on the job, it is probably because relatively few people have much of either.	______	______	______	______
14. One problem in asking for the ideas of subordinates is that their perspective is too limited for their suggestions to be of much practical value.	______	______	______	______
15. It is only human nature for people to try to do as little work as they can get away with.	______	______	______	______

Totals for columns ______ + ______ + ______ + ______ = ______

(×1) ______ + (×2) ______ + (×3) ______ + (×4) ______ + =

Grand Total ______

Source: Reprinted from the ORC Public Opinion Index, August, 1961. Copyright Opinion Research Corporation, 1961: used with permission.

Now answer these questions by checking the column for each statement that comes closest to your position. The test should take no more than three or four minutes.

Scoring and Meaning of the Test

1. Total the number of check marks in each column and insert these numbers in the appropriate blanks at the end of the test (Exhibit 2-1). Obviously, if you have not skipped any statements and if you have totaled correctly each column, the Totals for Columns row should add across to 15.

2. Next you should multiply whatever total you have for each column as follows: multiply your total in the Strongly Disagree column by one and write this figure below column one; multiply your total in the next column by 2 and write this figure below column 2; multiply the third column's answer by 3 and the fourth column's answer by 4 in like manner. (Remember, by the way, that any number multiplied by zero is still zero, even in the new mathematics!)
3. Now add up the four figures you just arrived at by multiplication. The sum of these four figures is your Grand Total. Again, if you have not made any mathematical errors, your answer is somewhere between 15 and 60.

To interpret your numerical score, it is necessary to consider Figure 2-1. The line A to D is intended to provide for all possible sets of assumptions regarding people and their work. Points from A to M represent various degrees of autocratic or authoritarian styles of management; M to D covers differing amounts of democratic or developmental supervision.

The theory here is that your set of assumptions about people and their work is what leads you to develop a certain style of management. The autocrat considers people as having little ambition and trying to avoid responsibility by wanting to be told what to do at all times. This leads the manager to assume the responsibility for setting objectives and to exercise close control to see that these objectives are carried out. It fosters a relationship in which subordinates are dependent and show relatively little self-expression or self-responsibility. In this sort of a climate the participative decision making of MBO finds little nourishment.

On the other hand, developmental supervision is based on the assumption that to challenge people with real opportunity can encourage them to excellence of performance. It is the result of looking upon people as accepting and even enjoying their work and eager to accept responsibility. It leads to participation in the setting up of objectives and to the exercise of broad control in such a way that people grow by monitoring

---

Figure 2-1 Styles of Supervision

STYLE	A Autocratic	M Developmental D
1. Often called.............	BOSS	LEADER
2. Motivates from..........	FEAR	INSPIRATION
3. Supervision is...........	CLOSE	GENERAL

themselves. It fosters a relationship in which subordinates can be independent and self-reliant, if their temperaments allow.

Notice how the actions of the individual manager will flow logically from attitude or assumptions about people and their capacity for development. Since autocrats believe that people dislike work and avoid it when they can, that they must be closely directed and controlled, that they are not interested in self-development, then they are prone to the following kinds of action:

- say little unless something is wrong
- be uninterested in the ideas of others
- decide what information people need
- change demands unexpectedly
- be sometimes hard to talk to
- discourage people from taking risks
- set objectives *for* subordinates
- unilaterally decide what indicates satisfactory performance

Conversely, since developmental managers believe that people accept and enjoy work, that they can direct and control themselves, that they accept and seek responsibility, their actions are likely to:

- consider ideas that conflict with their own
- allow a reasonable margin for error
- try to help others learn from their mistakes
- have consistently high expectations
- encourage people to reach in new directions
- help people understand the objectives of their jobs
- allow people to make their own commitments
- set objectives *with* people

It must be realized that it is rare to find one or the other style of management in the "pure state," as it were. Most of us fall somewhere along a line from the pure autocrat on the one hand to the pure developmental manager on the other. The individual circumstances surrounding any action can dictate what you will do at any given moment in time, but the general pattern of behavior you develop over time is what will place you on the continuum, either to the right or to the left of the midpoint. The key words in Figure 2-1 give at least a brief summary of the two opposite styles being considered.

1. If we are talking about an *autocratic* person, the one who cracks the whip, there is a small four-letter word, a polite four-letter word, that might be used to describe such a person. The word is *boss*. Why is *boss* appropriate? Because of the connotation behind it. You do not think of a pleasant person when you hear or use the word *boss;* to the contrary, you think of a firm taskmaster. On the other hand, what is a simple word to call a developmental kind of manager? How about *leader?* It's positive, and yet there is nothing harsh about it. As a matter of fact it seems to connote some empathy, enthusiasm, or self-confidence when you talk about a person as your leader. A leader is someone you *want* to follow, whereas the boss is someone you *have* to follow, like it or not.

2. Now how about their approach to getting things done? When bosses have a job to be done, how do they go about it in regard to giving instructions? Usually by barking orders. Or, if it is something not to be done, by forbidding. Or by using the "carrot" approach. So the boss motivates out of fear we say; relies on threats and rewards; orders and "no-nos"; that's the way to get things done. What do developmental-type managers do instead? They motivate by suggestion, by invitation, by persuasion.

3. Finally, the two types of managers use a different procedure in the daily supervision of the work of their people. The autocratic leader gets involved in all the details: tells people not only *what* to do, but *how* to do it, *when* to do it, *where* to do it, crosses every "t" and dots every "i," giving detailed instructions. This we call "close" supervision. The developmental supervisors, on the other hand, do not give the details of what, when, where, and how. They stimulate the use of initiative, delegate, encourage the thought process of the person doing the job, and thereby allow subordinates continuing opportunities to mature.

Now back to your score on the test. Before finding out what your score means, you should do one more thing. If the purpose of the test is to place you somewhere on the continuum from autocratic to developmental, where do you think your position will be? Do you think you will be somewhere to the left of the midpoint: that is, that you are somewhat autocratic in your method of handling people? If so, place an *A* somewhere on the line to the left of the midpoint indicating how far over you think you may be. Or, do you feel you are somewhere to the right of center; that is, that you are developmental to some degree or other in your normal handling of people? If so, place a *D* somewhere to the right of center indicating how far over you think you are.

According to those who devised this test, as borne out by the many groups who have subsequently taken it and about whom there was sufficient information to check validity and reliability, your score can be interpreted as follows: if you scored 39 or higher, you are probably autocratic;

if you scored 29 or less, you are probably developmental. The highest possible score was a 60—a pure autocrat; the lowest possible score is a 15—a pure democrat (no political inference meant!). If you scored between 29 and 39, you don't have strong leanings one way or the other.

What other use can be made of this exercise? Here are some suggestions as you continue your self-examination:

- Are you consistent? That is, does your score agree with your "guesstimate" of your position on the continuum? If you placed yourself on the "wrong" side of center, then you may be in trouble; you may not know enough about your own method of handling people, or at least you don't have the same image of yourself as others do, because your score on this projective test is probably the view others have of you.
- If you are way out at the autocratic end of the scale, that is, if you scored somewhere between 52 and 60, then you are probably in trouble. This means you have definite "high-handed" tendencies in dealing with people. You apparently feel that people do not have much initiative of their own, that they have to be watched very carefully, that they have nothing to contribute of value to a group endeavor, and that they are motivated primarily by selfishness. You are probably, therefore, control-oriented in directing their activities and will likely run into difficulty using MBO as a participative tool.
- If you are way out on the developmental end of the continuum, that is, you scored somewhere between 15 and 20, you may also be headed for trouble. Why? Because you apparently do not have sufficient sense of the need for controls. You are perhaps too permissive in your approach to people and might well be overly idealistic in terms of their response. In using MBO you may, therefore, tend to refrain from holding people accountable for achieving the standards agreed upon.
- Even if you scored in the middle, that is, 33 to 35 or thereabouts, you could have problems. It depends on how you got this score. If you checked some answers in the first column and some answers in the last column, so that the pluses offset the minuses as it were, trouble could result because you do not recognize the inconsistency of your responses. A careful reading of the 15 statements will indicate that all of them really say the same thing in a different way. So, at the very least, you should not strongly agree with some and then strongly disagree with others. Answers running down the middle two columns, even though they are labeled agree and disagree are really not inconsistent, given the rapidity of your response and the absence of a neutral position.

Question: With this as a background about you and your personal style, about where on the continuum in Figure 2-1 do you think we should plot MBO as a system of management? What numerical score do you think it would have? Why?

Answer:

You should have said that MBO belongs somewhere on the line between 29 and 20; not that the numbers really mean anything: they are simply a convenient way of illustrating that the philosophy of MBO carefully seeks a combination of two concepts that some people think are mutually exclusive. The first concept is that of *participative decision making:* MBO very definitely is for the purpose of decentralizing, delegating, and developing people in the organization through a sharing of the decision-making process. This is because of the commonly observed fact that when people have a say in making a decision, they are more likely to exert the energy it takes to accomplish what that decision entails. Through participation comes a degree of ownership of the decision, and that usually is the motivating force to get people to work hard to achieve the results of the decision. When those decisions deal with the very core of a person's job, it is absolutely essential that the individual feel some of that ownership of the decision as to what the job is intended to produce.

The second concept, or value, which keeps us from placing MBO further to the right side of the line, is *accountability*. When people share in the authority of making decisions, they have a responsibility to fulfill those decisions: they must be held accountable for whether or not the objectives they voluntarily impose upon themselves as a measure of doing the job well are accomplished.

Here is a common objection from many who do not really understand what the word *accountability* means: "But there are many things about my job that I cannot control, so I don't want to be held accountable for them." This is confusing *accountability* with *culpability.*[2] To be accountable for something means literally to be able to render an account, to be the one to explain what happened or what did not happen and why. It says nothing about whose fault it might be that some desired result did or did not materialize. To be completely candid about it, there are precious few of us who can literally control all variables that impact upon our results. There are always policies, environmental constraints, cooperation from others, economic considerations, information, and assumptions about both present and future, and so forth that have a lot to do with the success of our ventures. If we had to have control over all these before being able to make a commitment about our objectives, there would be very few valid objectives. But we might be able to give an account about what happened and how all these variables might impact our results. And we might decide ahead of time about what we might be expected to be able to influence if not control.

MBO seeks to pinpoint responsibility, but not in the sense of being on a witch hunt. We're not playing good guys and bad guys. We're not playing what Dr. Eric Berne calls the game "NIGY, SOB," in which one person waits around until the other fails to meet a commitment and then pounces on the already despondent failure.[3] You can make a commitment to an objective that you cannot control, and if the objective is not met, as long as there is a good explanation as to why you did not achieve it, if it was for reasons you were not expected to be able to influence, you have rendered an account and may not be guilty of anything. But at least you have brought the reasons to someone's attention so that effective action can be taken or decisions made to modify the objective if no one can effect the results.

Question: So the two values are what?
Answer:

The answer is participation and accountability. Now we need to turn our attention to procedures that will help us maintain the very delicate balance between these two. Starting in the next chapter we will begin to recommend steps to implement such a results-oriented system, and every recommendation we make will be for the purpose of protecting these two values. For in every instance we know of in which MBO did not help the hospital or the department, it was because of improper blending of both these values. In some instances MBO was seen as mainly a way to get people to make commitments, and once the commitment was made, it was held over people's heads like a club: all accountability and no participation, so it didn't work. In other instances, people were led to think that participation meant one long rap session after another seeking a decision that made everyone happy, without ever coming to closure as to who would be accountable for what in a nonthreatening way: all participation and no accountability, so again it didn't work.

SUMMARY

This chapter is designed to provide a link in our discussion of the theory and practice of MBO. It affords an opportunity to check our predisposition for the process involved in MBO. Unless the right climate of management prevails in the hospital or in the particular department we manage, the likelihood is that the system will flounder. Previous experience reveals that the system has not worked in situations in which the manager's style of leadership was not conducive to participative decision making.

If the test offered in this chapter or some other reliable method of checking out the managerial climate suggests that managers might not be likely to trust the judgment of subordinates, the best conclusion one should make regarding the installation of MBO is: wait. It *is* possible that an individual manager, or an entire company, might not be ready for MBO. To attempt to implement the system without the proper climate is to invite failure.

Such a situation calls for preliminary steps to improve the likelihood of success. This usually means management development programs geared at increasing responsibility at lower levels of management. It might also mean organization development interventions such as the introduction of responsibility accounting, the delegation of more authority to subordinate supervisors, deliberate use of more group approaches to problem solving and decision making, more effective use of committee structures, widening staff meetings and department head meetings to include more levels of supervision—these are among the techniques available and likely to be helpful in preparing the way for MBO.

NOTES

1. Harry Levinson, "Management by Whose Objectives?" *Harvard Business Review*, July–August, 1970, p. 125.
2. For a very intriguing discussion of how holding people accountable for their objectives is not necessarily being autocratic, see Larry Greiner, "What Managers Think of Participative Leadership," *Harvard Business Review*, March–April, 1973.
3. Eric Berne, *Games People Play* (Ballantine Books paperback edition, 1973), pp. 85–87.

Chapter 3

Installation of a Total System in the Hospital

Now we are ready to treat the steps in implementing a hospitalwide program of MBO. The purpose of this chapter is to set forth a model for a step-by-step approach to install the system, to offer advice about procedures that can be used at each step, and once again to offer examples drawn from the experience of hospitals currently using MBO.

THE DECISION TO INSTALL

The first basic decision to be made by the CEO of the hospital is whether the program is to be hospitalwide from the start. Some organizations have found it more effective in the long run to take a soft-sell approach and not to install the system in a given department until the managers in that department have asked for it. This seems to be a reasonable approach to follow in very large organizations, which might be even geographically decentralized. We discussed in Chapter 2 the importance of having a climate or preconditioning conducive to the philosophy of MBO in any size organization.

But it is our opinion that the case for modular implementation (i.e., department by department when each is ready) has been best argued when the program is viewed as a personnel department program or a training department program.[1] This is not the approach being recommended here. It has been our contention from the start that one of the major advantages of MBO to a hospital is the unification of so many different management backgrounds into a real team because of the adoption of a single philosophy and a single approach to planning, organizing, directing, motivating, and controlling. The modular method of installation would delay this unification. Other issues relative to the modular approach are briefly addressed in Chapter 18.

Further, we have viewed MBO as a potent force for pushing the decision-making process down through the organization, as something CEOs want to do as their way of managing other managers, not as "another training program." Unfortunately, where MBO has acquired the image of coming from or belonging to a staff office (personnel, education, management development/training), it has suffered from the same unenthusiastic response too often given to any project so labeled (e.g., the budget or performance appraisals). That is, they seem to be treated as an imposition on the line manager, an intrusion on his already busy day, an interruption in his real work, to be brushed aside as soon as possible "to get back to my job."

To avoid this reaction to MBO, the suggestion here is that CEOs make this their project. Emphasize the team-building aspect; get across the idea that "around here everyone is going to manage by objectives," as a way of managing, not as a training program. If some departments appear to be less ready than others, take some of the preparatory steps discussed in Chapter 2, remembering even then that it will always be necessary to expect more or less sophistication in the use of the system by different hospital managers, depending on individual competencies.

The main idea in this initial decision is to announce it widely. Following the principles of participative management discussed earlier, the CEO must involve the top administrative team in arriving at the decision. This itself will do much to ensure the correct response to the official decision. But to get all levels of managers really behind the program, it is advisable to create a little stir at the time of the announcement. Some hospitals have set aside a section of their main bulletin board (near the time-card clock, or in the employees' cafeteria), clearly marking it for MBO news, to stimulate hospitalwide interest. A sample of the sort of announcement placed on this board to announce MBO is seen in Exhibit 3-1. These efforts go a long way toward creating an environment in which "objectives" become a part of daily conversation among all workers.

The decision to install the program should also consider how *deeply* into the organization the program will go initially (as opposed to how *broadly*). Some CEOs find it more effective to limit the formal preparation and discussion of objectives to the administrative team and the department head levels the first time through. After these two levels of management have had a year's experience with the system, they usually feel a little more comfortable with the whole program and can take a more affirmative role in implementing it at lower levels of management within each department.

Figure 3-1 is the step-by-step process recommended to get the program established after the initial decision to install has been made. The three

Exhibit 3-1 Sample Bulletin Board Announcement

UPDATING OUR MANAGEMENT SYSTEM

It takes a lot of skills to provide the patient care we wish to provide for our community. We have those skills in the person of our employees, professional and nonprofessional alike.

It also takes a lot of coordinative effort on the part of managers to plan, direct and control the use of all these skills. Newer and better theories and techniques of doing the work of a supervisor are constantly being developed.

To help bring some of these improved management techniques to our hospital, we have retained professional management consultants. Starting on ________________ they will conduct a series of meetings with management and supervisory personnel in order to install a system called MANAGEMENT BY OBJECTIVES.

Making this system helpful to us will be *hard work*. But the payoff as already experienced in many industrial companies, governmental agencies, and other hospitals proves it is all worth the effort.

Your cooperation is requested in helping us use this approach to do a better job for our patients as well as for all employees.

WATCH THIS BOARD FOR FURTHER INFORMATION!

lines of activities correspond to the three basic levels of management in the typical hospital: top management, department head level, and supervisors within each department. Time is measured from left to right on the model. The precise length of time between activities is not very significant. What is important is that each level of management carry out its assigned steps before calling on subordinate levels to participate in the program. This is not just to give a good example but to provide the information needed at each successive level.

TOP MANAGEMENT TRAINING

Who should be included in the top management level? While it is recognized that the CEO and his/her associate and/or assistant administrators will be the ones most involved in using MBO as a daily management tool, it is strongly urged that the entire board of directors (trustees) participate in the initial learning experience. They will then be in a better position to use the management information system generated by the MBO program and might be less prone to want to superimpose their own reporting/

Figure 3-1 Steps for Installing the System Hospitalwide

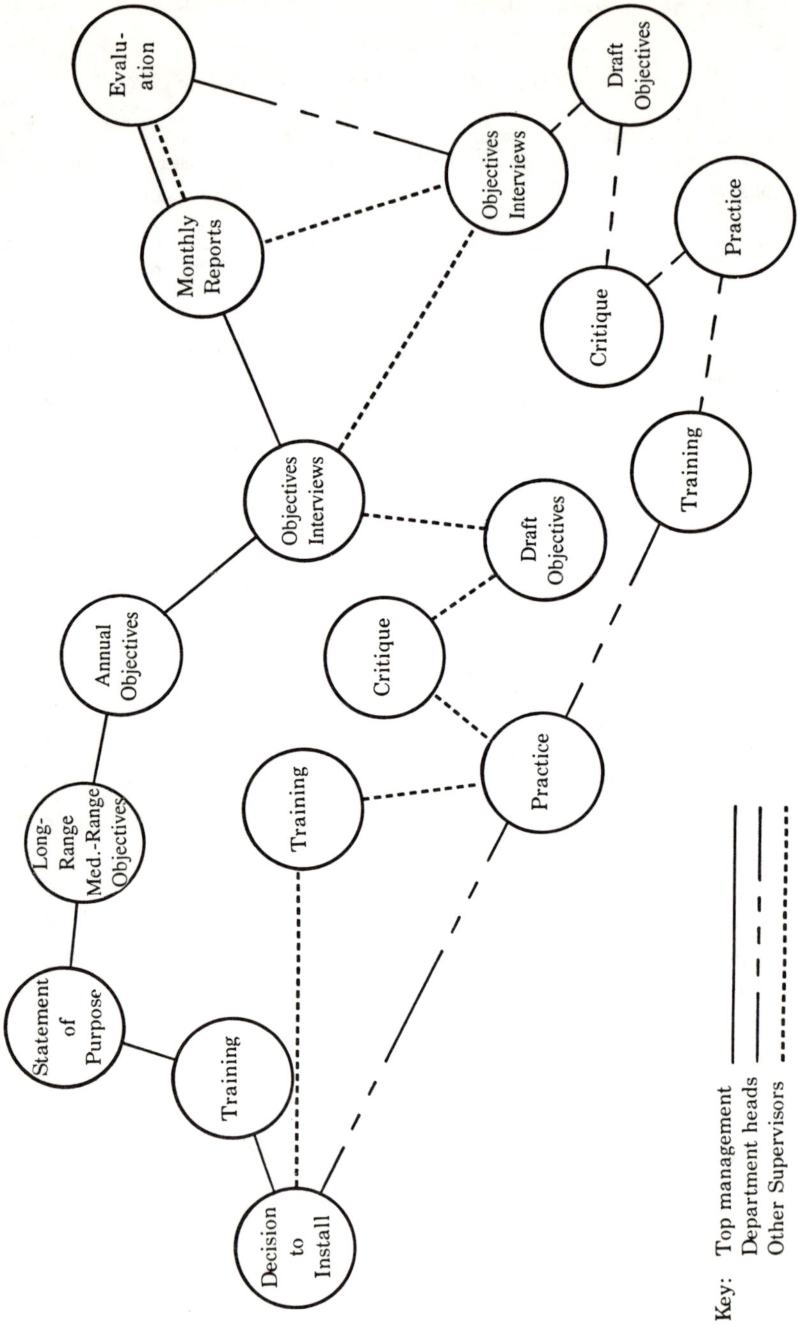

control devices on the hospital CEO. They will also find the emphasis on measurable results in keeping with their own desire to concentrate on outputs and not get involved in all the operational details of administration.

It is also a good idea to include representatives of the medical staff in the top administrative team when possible. The chief of staff or executive committee can often lend much needed support in implementing objectives later if they are invited to participate in setting priorities in the MBO program.

The first step after the decision to install should be some kind of training for the top administrative team. Since they must start the process at their level and since other managers will be taking their cue from what top management does, it is important that the top administrative team produce imitable results and understand their role in subsequent steps. If they expend the time and effort on learning the system, other managers will appreciate that this is not just another control program to obstruct middle and lower levels of management but one in which administration actively participates just as they will ask others to do. (This helps prevent the unanswerable comment most often heard from lower levels of managers when their training is held, "Too bad my boss isn't here to get this!")

The provision of training of some sort at every level as a first step is essential. A hospital CEO simply cannot learn about MBO (from a book, a seminar, a convention) and send a memo to all departments saying in effect that, commencing on such and such a date, "We're all going to manage by objectives!" As with most effective management tools, MBO requires an investment of time and effort to learn. The realization of how much time it takes to learn and then how much time it takes to do a good job in stating objectives is just as important as the appreciation of how much time MBO will save for the manager in the long run—time that will ultimately be used to manage instead of spinning wheels.[2]

The training for the top administrative team can be accomplished in a number of ways, but basically it will be either by attendance at some outside learning experience or by an in-house training program. Whichever route is chosen (and either can be effective), perhaps the best advice, in addition to being sure of the qualifications of the trainer, is to see that all members of top management hear the same message and engage in the same learning experience. If possible, it should be done as a group, rather than one or two individuals at a time. Two or three intensive days is really all we are talking about. There are three main reasons for this advice, which might seem obvious to readers who have participated in similar learning experiences.

1. MBO is not a precise science. There are as many different understandings of how to do it as there are persons who believe they have had success with it. While any of several successful approaches might work, trying to combine several usually negates them all. Therefore, it is best to have everyone get the same basic message.
2. Applying MBO to different environments is a special art. The hospital is going to use the system a little differently than will the manufacturing firm or the bank. If different hospital managers learn about MBO with several different types of other managers, they will undoubtedly come together with different perspectives of how useful it will be to them. While variety adds new insights, the commitment to gaining the benefits of the system could be hurt. Again, it is best to have everyone get the same basic message.
3. Later on, members of top management will have individual work in dealing with their own immediate subordinates, and a personalized approach will undoubtedly be helpful then. But the first work of the administrative team will be to work as a team on the over-all hospital purpose. Consequently, it is best to have everyone get the same basic message and at the same time, if possible.

Statement of Purpose

Much will be said in Chapter 5 about the distinction between the purpose, or reason for existence, and objectives. Our conclusion at that point will be that statements about high quality of patient care and the like are not good statements of objectives, but they still serve an important function. Hospital personnel are, by and large, very dedicated people. Hospital executives increasingly come to the health care field from other industries because of motivation (sometimes subconscious) to fulfill self-actualizing needs. They need to see their own personal commitments spelled out as part of the hospital's mission.

In addition, there is the organizational principle that structure flows from purpose—function follows form. Before you can begin stating measurable objectives, you should be clear as to ultimate purpose. In the hospital, this means reviewing and/or restating the corporate charter. It is the responsibility of the administrative team to be sure the statement of purpose is intelligible to all managers and that all objectives subsequently worked out are set in light of this purpose.

Chapter 5 will offer an instrument for involving the whole team (including board members and the medical staff) in coming up with such a statement of purpose as part of a needs analysis of the hospital. Our intent in Chapter 6 is to look at the whole model, step by step, and see how each activity ties in with the others in implementing the whole system. Therefore, it is sufficient at this point simply to give illustrations of the finished product—called by different people the *general mission* (example in Exhibit 3-2), statement of *philosophy* (example in Exhibit 3-3), the *purpose* (example in Exhibit 3-4), or the hospital *credo* (example in Exhibit 3-5).

In Chapter 5 we express our preference that a hospital's philosophy, credo, purpose, and role be combined into a comprehensive statement of mission, and the rationale behind this. Figure 5-1 illustrates the relation of these terms to one another.

Exhibit 3-2 Example Statement of General Mission

GENERAL MISSION

The fourfold purpose of ______________________ Hospital is to provide comprehensive, high quality patient care, to facilitate the educational process in medicine and allied fields, to provide health care services to the total community served by the hospital, and to encourage appropriate medical research. There are many important considerations affecting the attainment of each of these purposes, some of a material nature and others relatively intangible, but all pertinent to the establishment of a framework within which the general mission of the hospital can be carried out.

The provision of comprehensive, progressive, high quality patient care includes the concept of both in-patient and out-patient care, care for those with financial resources and for those without, and care provided to individuals without regard to race, color, or creed. It is limited of necessity by the financial resources that can be mobilized at a given time to carry out its programs.

The educational programs are designed to provide formal instruction and clinical experience to a variety of medical and paramedical programs. Inherent in these programs is a profound belief in the fact that such activities serve to improve the general level of health care provided by the hospital and carry out our responsibilities to replace ourselves, that is, to provide the doctors, nurses, and technicians of tomorrow. The establishment of formal approved, self-contained educational programs and affiliation with established schools, colleges, and universities both serve these dual practical needs.

Our community responsibilities extend far beyond our walls and require that we offer leadership and guidance as well as services to that community. These can take the form of internal services, such as the Avery Clinic or the Emergency Room, or the form of collaborative, cooperative effort with other hospitals, planning agencies, and community groups. They require us to provide direction in the development of new health care programs and methods of fulfilling community health care needs, including the creation of new organizational structures, where these might be required. We need to be responsive to the health care needs expressed by the community.

To acquire and hold on to a top-level, progressive medical staff requires that we encourage their active participation in clinical research activities in conjunction with universities, governmental agencies, voluntary agencies, and other recognized ethical sponsors of such activities. Protection of the patient's interests must be a paramount consideration in all such programs, and formal protections must be devised on his behalf.

Exhibit 3-2 continued

The successful achievement of our aims makes it imperative that we provide effective and efficient management at all administrative levels leading to delivery of health care services economically, without unnecessary waste or duplication. This requires constant efforts to improve the managerial process through training, upgrading, and ongoing programs directed toward improvement. It further requires sound fiscal operation on both a short-term and a long-term basis through planning, budgeting, and prudent fiscal management.

From a social point of view, it is important that we serve as a responsible employer and community force through development and administration of sound, progressive, and equitable personnel policies and salary schedules. We can further discharge this community responsibility by participating in programs designed to improve the quality and effectiveness of the health care field through cooperative action programs, assuming an active role in joint membership associations and supporting institutional and professional membership societies.

Finally, the continued success of any organization is dependent upon its ability to communicate, both internally and externally, its reasons for being, its accomplishments, and its future goals. These must be addressed to a diverse group of audiences including the general public, patients, employees, medical staff, the medical community at large, donors, and various voluntary and government agencies. In this manner, a broad base of understanding and support can be focused on providing the resources and the climate to accomplish the purposes for which we exist.

Exhibit 3-3 Sample Statement of Philosophy

____________________ Hospital believes that man, created in the image and likeness of God, is a unique combination of body, soul and mind. The concept of health, as applied in the hospital, goes beyond the borders of medicine. ____________________ Hospital firmly believes in man's right to health, his right to care when he is ill, and his right to die in dignity and peace.

Among the most valuable resources are human intelligence and ingenuity. Therefore, the best professional, para-professional and ancillary talent will be employed at ____________________ Hospital and will be placed in an environment which will facilitate proper utilization of knowledge, intellect and skill. The hospital will maintain a balanced compensation program for all employees clearly related to job requirements of skill, responsibility, education and experience, and will maintain working conditions that are safe, clean, attractive, and conducive to excellent patient care. The hospital will conduct its supervision so as to emphasize respect for the uniqueness and dignity of its employees.

Strong administrative direction is of paramount importance in providing the climate in which the specific and collective goals can be achieved within the parameters of good fiscal management. The operations of the hospital are to be led by a capable management group that will have the respect of the organization for its human approach to everyday problems, fairness and business ability.

Exhibit 3-3 continued

Education, for both patients and employees, is not a by-product, but a continual process whereby the staff will improve the quality of patient care, a process in which personal enrichment may be experienced. Support will be given to facilitate appropriate research.

The hospital, as a member of an Association of independent comprehensive health care facilities, will respond, through the health apostolate of the __________________ to the needs of the community and through its long-range planning effort will help identify those needs. __________________ Hospital will continue to develop and strengthen the services and programs that are unique to its operations.

The continued success of __________________ Hospital is dependent upon its ability to communicate, both internally and externally, its reasons for being, its accomplishments, and its future goals. These must be addressed to a diverse group of audiences including the general public, patients, employees, medical staff, Auxiliary, the medical community at large, donors, and various voluntary and government agencies.

Exhibit 3-4 Sample Organizational Purpose

The primary purpose of __________________ Osteopathic Hospital is to improve the quality of life by providing the environment for the best possible emergency, in-patient and out-patient care.

Through cooperative efforts of the Board of Trustees, medical staff, administration and employees, the hospital is committed to:

- Advancing and supporting the principles and practices of Osteopathic medicine with a major emphasis on the practice of family medicine.
- Operating efficiently and on a fiscally sound basis, both internally and through cooperation and shared services with area hospitals, institutions and agencies.
- Providing a safe, clean and attractive physical environment.
- Recognizing the total person as a human being with psychological and emotional needs, as well as physical, which will enable the sick and injured to recover with dignity and will alleviate the suffering of the terminally ill patient.
- Searching for better ways to provide Health Care; offering educational opportunities, to include training of physicians, providing a proper clinical setting for persons entering health care professions, continuing education programs for employees and medical staff, patient teaching and preventive health care programs in the community.
- Developing our human resources by providing an environment for individual growth, a fair and equitable wage program, equal employment opportunities, a productive atmosphere for labor-management relations and recognition of the values and efforts of volunteers.

Exhibit 3-5 Sample Statement of Credo

____________________ Hospital is a charitable health care institution which has existed since 1880 in Denver, serving the Rocky Mountain and its contiguous states in a tradition of excellence. The hospital is committed to be a leader and model for the innovative and creative delivery of health care practices and management.

The purposes of the Hospital are: (1) Promotion of good health concepts and practices in the community. (2) Support for medical and allied health education to improve the standards and availability of quality medical care. (3) The provision of medical care to the less fortunate, especially the elderly and indigent patient, without discrimination or discourtesy. (4) Promotion of the moral, spiritual, and ethical values of the dignity, freedom, and responsibility of people and families by the Episcopal Diocese of Colorado. (5) Medical and clinical research selectivity.

The Hospital will aggressively develop community services in response to identified needs in its service area. The Hospital resource complex will continue to provide primary medical care to metro Denver and tertiary care in the Rocky Mountain and Plains States. A special commitment to serving downtown Denver has been authorized. Clinical and specialized research will be supported in selected areas, e.g. gerontology.

The Hospital commits itself to the provision of institutional health care in a responsible manner as a member of the greater Denver and Rocky Mountain communities. Health services will be shared where unnecessary duplication would otherwise result, and affiliations and shared services contracts are encouraged in all service areas. Concomitantly, a reasonable return on investment will be required for the hospital to maintain its leadership role and quality facilities, equipment and human resources.

The Hospital will challenge other area health institutions in the public interest by developing and maintaining a highly competitive rate structure for its health services. Such competitive fees for services will enhance consumer opportunities to a greater extent than burdensome and costly regulation.

Corollary to its responsible community health care and promotive role, the Hospital will actively participate in community planning processes and ensure the appropriate utilization of its medical resources. Methods to ensure appropriate utilization shall include aggressive marketing, multi-institutional ventures and affiliations, creative and innovative structuring of programs to finance and deliver health care, cost-effective institutional performance and competitive fees for services.

The hospital's continuing ability to serve its patients is important to its staff, employees, and the general public. It is recognized that financial constraints exist on the amount of charitable care or research which the hospital may engage in without financial support from the community. The Hospital will, within its available resources and including philanthropic solicitations for support, demonstrate community leadership in meeting the health needs of the disadvantaged population. Services from volunteer groups and auxiliaries have aided in the development of the Hospital. The hospital recognizes a commitment to stimulate, maintain and improve opportunities for volunteers and auxiliaries in the institutional affairs.

Employees of the hospital often are the hospital's most effective goodwill ambassadors to the general community. The hospital's recognition of their vital role in health care mandates the provision of fair wages and remuneration for services, high competency standards and skills development training and inservice education, the promotion of job satisfaction and the offer of competitive job benefits. A commitment to affirmative action in the selection and development of staff is included in the hospital's role as an institutional health services leader.

Exhibit 3-5 continued

The hospital believes in and supports the involvement of all segments of the hospital family in the development of the policies and practices which ensure the continued growth of the institution, the guidance and support of its Board of Managers, the interest and commitment of the medical staff, the dedication of its employees, the concern and wishes of patients and their families, the contributed time and services of volunteers, and the invaluable bequests and grants of community donors.

As the new decade indicates a time of change for health care institutions in our community, the challenge for ____________________ Hospital shall be to maintain the excellence which exists while pursuing appropriate resource utilization and multi-institutional affiliations to enhance the promotion of high quality health care in the Rocky Mountain and Plains region.

Long-Range and Medium-Range Objectives

The next step in implementing MBO is for the administrative team to review and/or prepare statements of objectives that go beyond a single year's operation. Sometimes it is helpful to distinguish between long-range objectives and medium-range objectives. The former are most often understood today to encompass anything that might take five years or more to accomplish. (Until the 1960s long-range planning committees were wont to be thinking in terms of 10 to 25 years. While we do not mean to deny the importance of having "visionaries" to dream about the distant future, we call attention to the trend among planners in most industries to considerably shorten the concept of long-range to five to ten years.)[3]

Most hospitals or hospital boards have a long-range planning committee. Most often the fruit of their work is a rather lengthy document incorporating statements of philosophy, strategies, fund-raising plans, and the like. The job for top management is to reduce such a document to the essential result statements, which describe answers to the question: "Where do we want to be—in several key areas of concern—five years from now?" Some long-range committees get bogged down trying to finalize their work. Often it will be found this is due not to lack of agreement on the final results but due to disagreement on the tactics to be used to obtain those objectives, with professional standards, personalities, or other factors really causing the hang-up. A review of work to date can succeed in breaking the log-jam if it is made clear that only results are to be incorporated into the long-range objectives, not the strategies.

Medium-range objectives, likewise, are understood here to incorporate results that take longer than one year to achieve but less than five years. It is not always necessary to have these two groups of objectives separately stated. But recognition should be given to the fact that although some results will not be accomplished in the present operational period, some effort will be required in the present period if the objective is to be ultimately achieved.

Chapter 5 will offer a series of probing questions in key areas of concern to help top management come up with the answers for the long- and medium-range objectives. But again our purpose in this chapter is to see how all the steps in implementing the system tie together, so it will suffice here to give some examples of what some long-range and medium-range objectives might look like. Exhibits 3-6 and 3-7 illustrate each type.

It will be seen at once that these results statements are not as specific in their measurability as are the examples in this chapter covering the present period of operations. Yet they are precise enough to fulfill the function of "letting us know when we get where we want to get" (a goal line). They do describe "the degree and direction of change from the present," as we will define any objective in Chapter 6.

Exhibit 3-6 Sample Long-Range Objectives

- Establishment of this hospital as not only an acute care facility, but also a medical center for this metropolitan area, with consequent emphasis on medical education and research.
- Consolidation of our services with those of other hospitals in our Area Planning District so that we do not duplicate services (and expenses) unnecessarily.
- Establishment of a long range statistical data base (population figures, economic data, highway plans, etc.) to enable the hospital to always have realistic and up-to-date long range plans.
- Gradual implementation of a policy of having the chief of each medical department (Medicine, Surgery, OB-Gyn, etc.) be paid hospital employees.
- Relocation of the hospital to a new location available to the people we serve where we can provide ________ more beds and ____________________ new services.
- Merger of our hospital with ____________ Hospital to provide one comprehensive health care facility for the people of this community with lower combined operating costs.
- Implementation of the "holding company" concept under which we join four smaller hospitals in providing one central administration for five institutions.
- From operations, funding 50 percent of depreciation for long term capital development.
- Generation of 3 to 5 percent net gain as a percentage of gross revenue each year.
- Reduction of operating deficit of our Clinic to $____________ by the development of outside sources of funds for support of this program.
- Development of a community relations program aimed at providing as many services for the community as are identified by community representatives and offering no services that are not seen by them as appropriate.

Exhibit 3-7 Sample Medium-Range Objectives

- Phasing out of our OB department in favor of ________________ Hospital, while they phase out their pediatric facilities in favor of us.
- Revised budget system to involve all department heads in the preparation of their budgets (capital and operating) with consequent financial information being shared with them.
- Development of a total management information system, using latest computer system and comparison with appropriate comparable hospitals, as a basis for tracking our own performance against our own objectives.
- Orderly transition into new building upon its completion.
- Establishment of administrative connection with nearby nursing homes to ensure place to transfer our patients when appropriate.
- Participation in feasibility study of centralized laundry facility.
- Erection of a 400-car parking structure on our property.
- Completion of a building fund drive to net $__________ within the next 36 months.
- Acquisition of grant from the federal government to permit implementation of at least two paramedical training programs.
- Initiation of construction of medical office building adjacent to our hospital, with ownership of same, vested in someone else.
- Completion of a skills inventory of all management staff in the several hospitals included in our corporation, to identify the quantity, quality and marketability of our personnel and the areas where back-up people are needed.
- Completion of micro-filming of all charts not on unit-record system.

Annually these long-range and medium-range objectives should be reviewed, and the question again asked, "Is this where we wish to be five years from now?" In this way they become not any given five-year period's objectives, but a kind of rolling five-year plan, adding another year to the far end with the passage of each new year.

Annual Objectives for the Hospital

Having reviewed the organization's purpose and long-range objectives, top management is now ready to set annual objectives. These will be seen as answers to the question: "If we are to carry out our purpose and get where we want to be five years from now, what must we accomplish this year, as a part of the overall plan?"

It is important to recall the use to be made of the list of hospital objectives. First of all, that will be used to evaluate whether the hospital is being managed adequately. Those objectives are the criteria for judging the competence of the management team of the hospital, and in particular the hospital CEO. In a true sense, they are *his/her* objectives. Therefore, they should include the important items for the board and the public to judge whether the CEO is properly doing his/her job. It should include their priorities for his/her guidance.

Since the CEO's job probably includes routine responsibilities, problem areas, and innovations, the list of objectives should include all three categories. (This will also serve as a model for other managers when it comes time for them to list their objectives.)

But the hospital CEO delegates the implementation of most responsibilities to various other hospital managers.[4] They will take the list of hospital objectives and use them as a point of reference for setting their own objectives. Therefore, the second use of the hospital objectives is to provide a cue to others as to the response expected from them. The complete list, then, must be broad enough to indicate priorities for major departments.

Herein lies one of the most critical pressure points for a viable MBO system. The hospital list must set true priorities for things to be carried out within departments yet not interfere with the managerial autonomy of the department head. It must set broad guidelines and leave room for operating within those parameters. Hospital CEOs must give directions to their subordinates and not preempt their decision-making prerogatives. How can one do this?

The following sequence of events has been found helpful in some hospitals as a way of involving department heads in determining the hospital objectives so they are not imposed from above, yet they truly can give the direction called for.

1. Hospital CEOs identify what they believe to be the key results areas, which should be included on the hospital list of objectives. They might arrive at this list by a needs analysis tool (such as described in Chapter 6), by consulting a checklist of top management concerns (e.g., as found in Peter Drucker, *The Practice of Management*), by calling to mind points covered in board meetings, by reviewing results of the last visit of the Joint Commission on Accreditation, and so forth. They give this list to key managers at the department head level with an invitation to join in a discussion of the indicators of success and specific numbers appropriate for the ensuing year. They are pointing to areas of concern without prejudging how much progress can be made in these areas and without consultation with those who will have to accomplish the results.
2. Hospital CEOs conduct a meeting with those department heads. In attendance should be major department heads and the top manage-

ment team. (As a rule of thumb, it is difficult to do this effectively if the number exceeds ten or so persons. Only as a "for instance," the list might include: chairman of the board, hospital CEO, two to three associate or assistant administrators, nursing service or patient care director, controller, personnel manager, chief of medical staff, director of laboratories, radiologist, director of development/public relations, director of buildings and grounds.) The purpose of this meeting is to respond to the list of key results areas: to suggest indicators of success, to recommend specific levels of achievement to be aimed at, and to offer additions or deletions from the list—all based on what the entire group believes to be realistic in the knowledge they have to implement the list. The dynamics of such a meeting often involve such things as:

- one or more managers will learn how important it is to others for them to raise or lower sights on a target of performance in their own department
- one or more managers will find that some pet project simply is not considered high priority on a hospitalwide basis
- one or more managers learn how strongly others are counting on them to achieve some goal because of its implications on other departments
- all managers begin to start thinking like the head of the organization by broadening their perspective

3. Hospital CEOs reflect on the recommendations given and do their best to reconcile these with other sources of information/pressures available. They consider demands and advice of the board, of third-party payers, of regulatory agencies, of community representatives and area planning councils, of financial backers and lenders, of professional groups, physicians, patients, and countless other sources. They do what is possible to blend all these (sometimes) conflicting inputs to the planning process and finalize the objectives to which they wish to commit the institution. These are *their* objectives!
4. Hospital CEOs communicate the finalized list of hospital objectives to the staff. In some cases they have to convince the board to be more realistic in what it can expect. In other cases it's a matter of selling the staff on the importance of raising their sights and inviting them to respond to a challenge they might not have recommended but that has become necessary for such and such reasons. Here the important thing is to give the reasons for any changes in the recommendations given. This is best done in a meeting, rather than by written memo only. The finalized list ought to be distributed to all

participants in the MBO system and explained in person to all department heads. Here the number in attendance can be larger than in point two above because more persons may be involved in implementing the list and the communications here is more top-down than bottom-up.

Figure 3-2 graphically displays the four events just described and shows how they lead to an invitation to each department head to respond (Step 5) by setting objectives to implement hospital objectives. Exhibit 3-8 illustrates the three categories of hospital annual objectives. Here it will be seen that the institution's objectives must be as precisely measurable as anyone else's.

TRAINING FOR DEPARTMENT HEADS

Somewhere between the review of long-range objectives and the involvement of key department heads in setting the hospital's annual objectives, training ought to be provided for department heads. This orientation will be necessary if department heads are to be effective in helping top management set meaningful, measurable, and communicable objectives. Without it, the tendency will be for such persons to lapse into discussion of philosophy. One way used at times is to include department heads in the initial training for top management, especially if training is done in-house.

But the principal work of department heads is to be in the formulation of their own departmental objectives, so their training ought to focus more immediately on setting objectives at that level. The complete preparation recommended for department heads includes formal training, practice on their own, and an opportunity for critiquing of their initial efforts. Most hospital managers are accustomed to a type of inservice that includes input → practice → demonstration. They will respond positively to a method of training that explains how to set objectives, gives them a chance to experiment on their own "where it doesn't really count," and then reinforces the practice by personal assistance and tutoring during a critique session.

We have provided such training in two different ways, which the reader might wish to consider. A group of 25 or so hospital managers can be completely prepared to use MBO in a two- or three-day seminar. Where a hospital is large enough to provide adequate coverage of the floor while managers are in training for such a length of time, this is the preferable approach. A combination of lecture, example, practice, and demonstra-

Figure 3-2 Events in Setting Annual Objectives

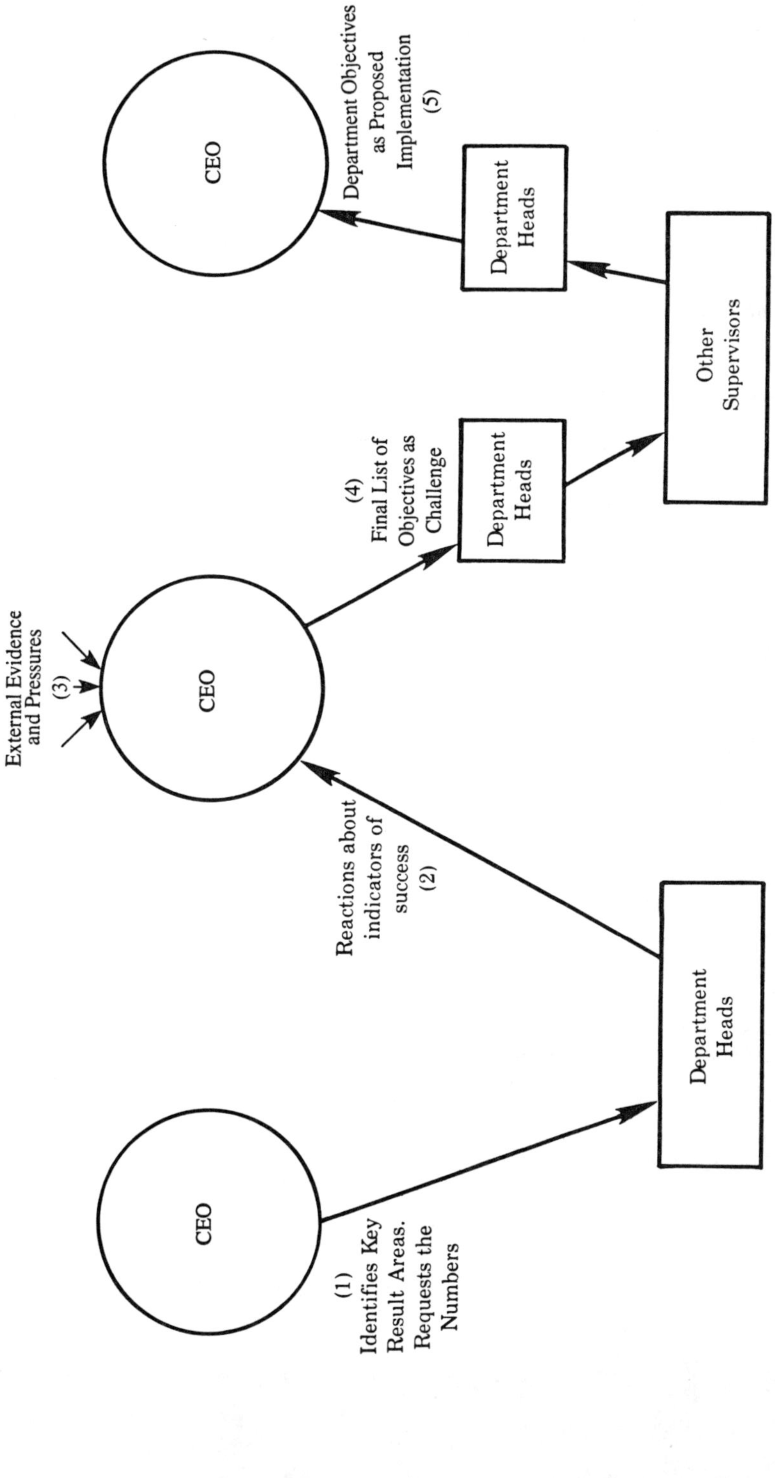

Exhibit 3-8 Sample Hospital Annual Objectives

Key Result Area	*Indicator of Success*	*Minimum Acceptable (Worst)*	*Expected Average*	*Maximum Probable (Best)*
Daily discharges	Percent accomplished by 11 A.M. daily	90%	92%	95%
Inventory of expendable supplies	Percent of previous year's on hand each department	90%	85%	80%
Maintenance of standards for accreditation	Number of departments meeting or exceeding those set by Joint Commission (out of 24)	18	20	22
Operating costs	Percent reduction across all departments over last year	5%	6%	7%
Personnel administration	Turnover of full time equivalents	40%	35%	30%
	Number of departments completing review of job descriptions (out of 24)	20	22	24
Productivity	Total number patient days divided by total number of FTEs	11.0	11.6	12.1
	Average patient stay (number of days)	8.6	8.4	8.2
Occupancy rate	All in-patient beds	91%	93%	94%
Accounts receivable	Outstanding by end of fiscal year	$700M	$600M	$550M
	Percent aged 6 months	8%	6%	4%
Establishment of MBO program	Number of departments completing goals, interviews, and monthly reports all year	20	22	24
New residency in pediatrics	Date opened	Feb 1	Jan 1	Dec 1
	Increased occupancy by year end	20%	25%	30%

tion can be worked into the two to three days. Immersion in the program is always best. (This assumes the program is seen as a step in the installation of the system, not as just another training program.) Where there cannot be the luxury of such an extended time off the floor, it is possible to do the same job by dividing the time into a half-day input, a couple of hours private application to practice, and another half-day critique session for groups up to 25.

Whichever method is chosen, it is essential that time be devoted to training department heads. Then they should be included in the final communication meeting with administration to become aware of the hospital's overall objectives. They should have a copy of what top management has prepared so far: statement of purpose, long-range and medium-range goals, and annual objectives for the whole institution. Now they are ready to prepare their own department objectives.

Drafting Departmental Objectives

It will be recalled that Chapter 2 emphasized the participative process as a touchstone of effective MBO. Perhaps the major proof of participation comes in the request for each department head to be the one to first put pencil to paper in drafting departmental objectives.

Top management has at this point provided all the help needed to do a good job: training in how to do it and guidelines in the shape of hospital objectives. The department head should respond to the hospital list the way anyone reacts to a challenge. The hospital objectives define the ideal of a well-managed institution. The department head should begin by asking "Are there any objectives on the hospital list I am primarily responsible for?" (It is hoped that the earlier discussion meeting regarding hospital objectives flagged all such objectives for each department head, so they would not miss any cue meant for them.) "Are there any objectives on the hospital list that call upon me to contribute some portion of the results?"

Taking Exhibit 3-8 as the objectives of a hypothetical hospital, the controller or business office manager would undoubtedly see the item referring to accounts receivable and would recognize that this must become a high priority item on his/her list, since it obviously falls within his/her area of responsibility. The controller or business office manager would also see the item concerning operating costs, calling on all departments to make a reduction, and would know that this must also be on his/her list somewhere, as he/she must make a contribution to this objective along with all other department heads. (There are others on the same list.)

But this is only the start of the list. Now the department heads must ask as regards their departments the same kind of questions the hospital CEOs asked themselves about the entire hospital. Within their departments, they are responsible for routine operations, for solving problems, and for improving performance by innovation. They should then make a list of key results areas and choose for each indicators of success and statements of results expected in all three categories. The many examples worked out in succeeding chapters will be helpful to department heads.

To check the completeness of this list of objectives, the department head might examine these points:

- If I were the hospital CEO, which key results areas in this department would I wish to monitor on an ongoing basis to be sure the department was under control? The department list is to be used by the CEO to check performance in the department and therefore should not include the minutiae but only the overall results. These are the department head's personal objectives, not the detail of all his/her people.
- As department head, have I given all my key people something on which to hang their hat? Can they find their cue in the list of departmental objectives? If not, perhaps the objectives are not broad enough.
- Before I go to the CEO and commit my department to these objectives, have I checked out what I plan to do with my key people? Do I have their ideas? It will be embarrassing to set an objective with the CEO and then find out my people cannot accomplish it.

This last point is another crucial pressure point for participative management in making MBO work. Department heads might wish within their departments to use the same approach recommended to the hospital CEO for the hospital annual objectives. That is, they may wish to feed their people some key results areas and invite their response as to the indicators of success and the actual numbers (results) before finalizing the draft for discussion with the CEO. They should avoid, however, the approach of *simply* getting the objectives of their people one by one, tying a rubber band around all, and bringing the package to the CEO as department objectives—without any work on their part. Such an approach is soon found to be unworthy of the department heads under questioning by the administrator.

Department Objective-Setting Interviews

Next come the one-on-one objective-setting interviews between each department head and his/her administrative superior. The rationale for these interviews and suggestions for conducting them will be treated at length in Chapter 7 in discussing how MBO works for individual managers.

A schedule for these interviews should be prepared in such a way that they are all accomplished in a relatively short span of time, say one calendar week. They take only about one hour each and, depending on the span of control, should not tie down any top management person for too many hours. Having a master schedule for them will enhance the likelihood that they will be accomplished. Confining them to a short time frame, such as one week, will make it possible to have a department head meeting shortly thereafter for the purpose of acquainting all departments with the objectives of each department and thus reinforce the need for mutual assistance. This latter has been the lesson from programs so far wherein evaluation of the use of MBO reveals some discontent that "I don't feel I know enough about mine!"

The final step relative to departmental objectives is providing copies of them to all subordinates within a given department. The departmental objectives become what we call *common* objectives for people at lower levels along with the hospital objectives.

TRAINING FOR OTHER SUPERVISORS

The third level of management on Figure 3-1 concerns supervisors within each department. In the typical hospital, it doesn't help much to identify fourth or fifth level persons (even though a department such as nursing service might well have fourth or fifth level persons).

At this level we simply repeat the basic training → practice → critique sessions as preparation for participation in the program. The length of time for training of this level supervisor is usually reduced in light of the reduced expectations mentioned in the next subsection.

Group training and critique usually realize many fringe benefits, such as greater appreciation for closer interdepartmental cooperation. In many hospitals supervisors at this level just do not customarily have the opportunity of discussing mutual concerns, and the MBO program often stimulates a round of sharing of information among such supervisors, which is never forgotten.

Drafting Objectives within Each Department

Supervisors are next invited by their respective department heads to prepare a draft of a statement of objectives to which they wish to commit themselves as a part of implementing hospital and departmental objectives. They now have the training in how to do it and should have copies of common objectives from which to take their cue.

They should start putting together their list as the department head did. They should begin with whatever they can see of the common objectives that fall to them directly or jointly with someone else. Such items are always high in priority on their list. But the list should not stop there. Supervisors go on to identify other results areas for which they are responsible.

What is happening in the whole organization is the building of a pyramid of objectives, where the base becomes quite broad by the time first-line supervision is reached. As seen in Figure 3-3, the original 15 or so hospital objectives can become several hundred as department heads find the 1 or 2 hospital objectives involving each of them and adding until they have maybe 10 to 15, and then supervisors begin with the 1 or 2 involving each of them and adding until they each have 6 to 8. (These numbers can be considered safe rule-of-thumb norms.)

Supervisor Objective-Setting Interviews

Next should come another round of one-on-one objective-setting interviews between supervisors and their department heads. Everything said about these interviews above applies at this level as well.

The output of such interviews should be written objectives, commitments between each superior-subordinate matched pair. Normally, copies of these objectives are not channeled above the department level. To do so invites supervisors to begin to deal directly with top management and short-circuit the chain of command, which may sound stuffy and archaic, but is still good organization theory if delegation of authority to department heads is to mean anything.

MONTHLY REPORTS

At this point the system is installed, and all that remains is its maintenance. It was mentioned earlier that feedback or constant monitoring of progress toward accomplishing objectives was as essential a part of MBO as the original setting of objectives. Yet many programs in hospitals and elsewhere get a great kick-off and then are left to die for lack of follow-up.

The first kind of follow-up recommended is a management information system, which automatically provides information for the manager to monitor progress and report that progress to others. Hence, in Figure 3-1, all three levels of management are seen converging at the point of these monthly reports.

Figure 3-3 Multiplication of Objectives as Each Level of Management Takes Cue from Above and Adds to Total

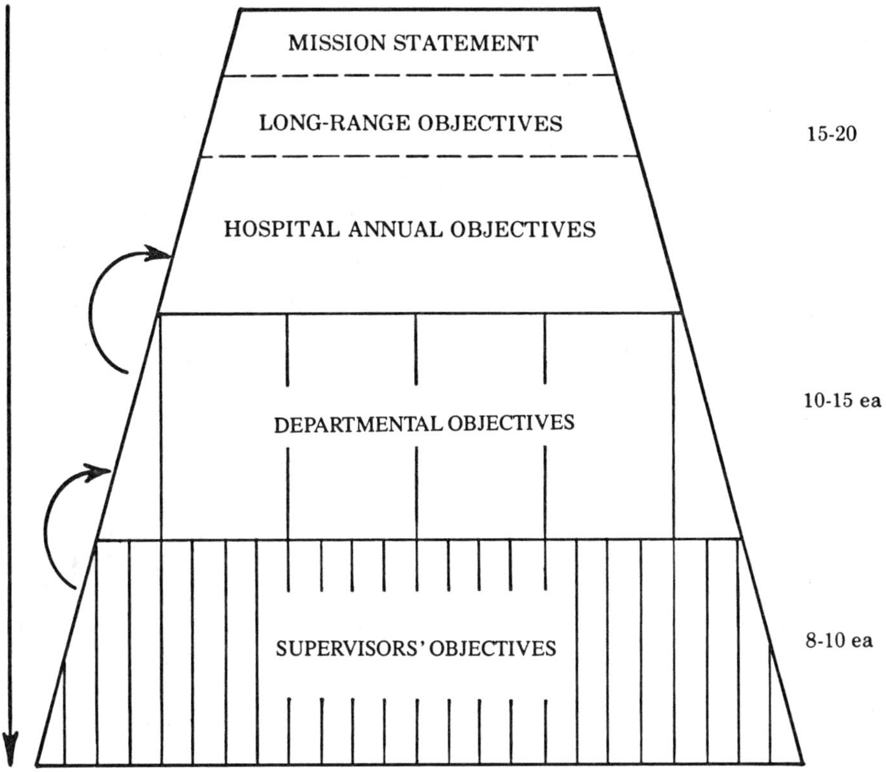

The statistics for tracking progress on routine objectives ought to be a byproduct of the routine management control system used by the hospital. Responsibility accounting means managers must be provided periodic financial information so they can see whether they are conforming to their budget. So also the personnel office, the controller's office, the data processing office, and all staff offices where appropriate information is collected and maintained should be geared to provide management information not only to the hospital CEO and the board but also to all managers so they can check their own performance in achieving objectives.

The integration of your MIS and MBO ought to be obvious. MBO cannot be a real system of management as proposed throughout this book unless the hospital's data base and periodic reporting system provide accurate and up-to-date information upon which managers can rely to make prudent judgments and decisions. It will be seen in subsequent chapters that the presence of such a data base will itself suggest opportunities for objective-setting.

In turn, this means all managers must provide the information needed for such reports. Most hospitals already have a routine of monthly statistical reports indicating procedures performed, meals served, laundry washed, and the like. It has been found feasible for department heads to add a small section to this monthly report entitled "Progress on Other Objectives" to report, using the exception principle, on matters not covered in the basic statistics. This information can then be collected and summarized in monthly statements to help top management keep track of progress on hospital objectives or departmental objectives, as needs warrant. An example of such summary reports is illustrated in Exhibit 3-9.

A second kind of follow-up about accomplishment of goals can best be handled by the appointment of a coordinator of MBO. This position, which is almost an essential in a large industrial organization, has been found to be of almost equal necessity as a part-time assignment for someone on the administrative team of a hospital.[5] A recommended brief job description for such a person emphasizes that this is not a position of decision-making authority, but more of a staff job to "bird-dog" and remind people of their responsibilities under the MBO program when a deadline for something is near. This would include such things as putting together the schedule for one-on-one interviews, designing monthly report forms, calling managers to see if they have done what they said

Exhibit 3-9 Sample Objectives Report

Name ______________________ Date ____________
Department ______________________ Period Covered ____________

Objective No.	*Negotiated Results*	*Actual Results*	*Comments*
(Just list the number, such as 1-a, 2-c, etc.)	(State the level intended by this time of the year)	(State the actual level at this time)	(State any explanation or suggestion, such as raising level, lowering level, changing indicator, trying new actions, deleting objective.)

Exhibit 3-10 Job Description

Title: Coordinator of MBO
Supervisor: CEO
Date:

Basic function: Under the direction of the hospital executive team—coordinates the training, utilization, and review of the hospitalwide system of management known as MBO for the purpose of integrating planning, improving superior-subordinate communications, and practicing participative decision making among all supervisory personnel.

Principal responsibilities:

1. Provides training opportunities for all new supervisory or management personnel, either in-house or at an outside location where MBO is taught competently.
2. Maintains ongoing interest in this system of management by periodic review of basic principles or discussion of examples of group meetings in the house organ, on the bulletin board, etc.
3. Gives individual tutoring, where needed, as an internal consultant for those requesting help in preparing objectives.
4. Prepares annual timetable for preparation and review of objectives at all levels.
5. Designs, distributes, and explains simple forms for the recording of objectives and reporting of progress in accomplishing them.
6. Follows up to ensure that objective-setting interviews between superior-subordinate matched pairs take place as scheduled.
7. Collects master file of objectives through department head level for the executive team and others as deemed appropriate.
8. Maintains "tickler file" on significant dates shown on various objectives and follows up with inquiries on said dates about results.
9. Creatively stimulates desire on part of all managers to achieve objectives through monthly reporting system.
10. Periodically fosters use of problem-solving model to build interdepartmental cooperation.
11. In all the above, works closely with line managers about objectives of their subordinates. THIS IS A *STAFF POSITION*.

they would do by promised dates, and so on. Exhibit 3-10 is a sample job description for such a position.

EVALUATION

The word evaluation here refers to the whole system of MBO, as well as to the performance of each manager in meeting objectives. Performance appraisal as such deserves its own separate chapter (see Chapter 16). As for the MBO program, the inference here is that the system should meet its objectives or be discarded. After the hospital has been using MBO for a reasonable length of time (two to three years) and assuming implementation at all levels of management, it should be formally evaluated.

The program was introduced as a tool of management intended to bring about certain benefits, described above as improved planning, improved superior-subordinate communications, improved motivation, and especially improved performance on the job. These ought to be the criteria for examining the worth of MBO to the organization after some period of working with it.

Chapter 19 contains a summary of the findings of a series of MBO usefulness surveys we conducted at several hospitals implementing MBO according to the steps outlined in this chapter; it might give some indication to the reader as to expected levels of satisfaction among hospital managers.

In our experience in evaluating systems of MBO, such an event not only revitalizes the program but also uncovers a host of feelings about the management of the organization. The evaluation has been likened at times to an attitude survey.

In the majority of cases, deficiencies in the program are readily identified, and corrective action instituted. At best, this has meant a more effective management team for the hospital and greater satisfaction with adoption of MBO in the first place. At worst, there have been occasions in which our honest advice to the hospital was "throw out the system" because it was not working, nor was there reason to believe it would in the near term. But, *do* something about the situation preventing it from working.

SUMMARY

This chapter has outlined a step-by-step model for the implementation of a full-blown system of MBO. It stressed the necessity of providing necessary preparation or orientation of managers to the philosophy and techniques of MBO before asking them to set objectives. It has followed the diverse responsibilities of three levels of management in implementing the system. It has called attention to two possible kinds of in-house support for the program: training personnel or an MBO coordinator. The importance of developing a satisfactory MIS to provide feedback on the progress in achieving objectives was also stressed.

As we now proceed into the two chapters of Part II, The Strategic Planning Part of MBO, we will examine the background and present status of planning in hospitals, as well as develop a comprehensive step-by-step process in preparing a long-range master plan for your hospital.

Succeeding chapters provide further helpful guidelines for each level of management as well as more examples of the sort of results that can be generated by each.

NOTES

1. cf John B. Lasagna, "Make Your MBO Pragmatic," *Harvard Business Review*, November–December 1971, p. 64.
2. F.D. Barrett, "The MBO Time Trip," *The Canadian Business Quarterly* (Autumn 1972): 42 ff.
3. Herman Kahn and B. Bruce Briggs, *Things to Come* (New York: MacMillan Co., 1972).
4. Arthur X. Deegan, II and Thomas R. O'Donovan, "How Much Authority Should the Administrator Delegate?", *The Modern Hospital*, October 1964, p. 94.
5. Gary D. Cardiff, "MBO—It *Will* Work in a Hospital Setting," *Hospital Administration in Canada*, November 1970, p. 23.

Part II

The Strategic Planning Part of MBO

Chapter 4

Growing Importance of Planning in Hospitals

BACKGROUND: HISTORICAL PERSPECTIVE

Development of comprehensive strategic planning programs by hospitals is the only way to survive external pressures that are continuing to control hospital expenditures and to contain operational revenues and capital formation of health care organizations. A sound planning process is the major effective force within hospitals to meet such challenges. In the months and years ahead hospital survival will depend upon sound planning today.

Up until a few years ago, long-range planning in some hospitals consisted of administrators and boards evaluating physician requests for equipment and how many new beds should be added. These were valid activities that needed to be addressed, but the difference between then and now is that planning has taken on a far greater dimension.

Planning is both an ongoing process and a learning process. As an ongoing process, planning starts by having the key members of your hospital family (board, administration, medical staff) make decisions regarding who you are and what you are about. Next you develop a comprehensive description and analysis of the external and internal environment in which your institution exists. Pertinent data must be gathered and interpreted, as will be described in detail later. A statement of issues and problems is then prepared. This now forms the basis for the formulation of your overall hospital objectives. Then comes programmatic planning, an evaluation process that is also ongoing, and the cycle repeats and continues, as does the progress of your hospital.

As a learning process, planning does not result in merely a good written document. The heart of planning is the ''jelling'' of all the members of the hospital family, including the community. In this way there is total support for the programs that will be developed in the master plan. Planning is a process whereby the entire future of your hospital has a better chance of being fulfilled. We have already referred to the importance of making decisions regarding who you are and what you are about. Unless you know yourselves thoroughly, inside and out, there is no way that you can begin to plan for your future.

The planning process at your hospital should cover all of the following:

1. the mission (or credo) of your hospital
2. carefully prepared overall administrative objectives, as well as sound departmental objectives
3. carefully prioritized programmatic planning (Should you be providing obstetric and pediatric services? Should you develop programs in oncology, high voltage radiation therapy, CT scanning?)
4. a comprehensive data base for planning (internally generated)
5. a successful public relations program (How's your image?)
6. formulation of sound marketing strategies (assess your competition)[1]
7. facilities planning (gearing up your plant to carry out programs and remodeling to meet new codes as they come up)
8. cooperative planning with area health care providers, health systems agencies (HSAs), and state health department certificate-of-need realities
9. medical staff recruitment as appropriate (How can you become the physician's hospital of choice?)
10. master plan of fund endowment and grantsmanship

Effective planning requires intelligence, time, and a commitment of resources. Planning never ends, and the long-range master plan is never completed. Benefits from sound planning may be slow in coming, but such benefits will never occur without building a solid foundation for planning. One of the major benefits of planning is the planning process itself. The entire hospital and its community must be integrated in order to produce a workable and acceptable plan. The importance of teamwork and the vital significance of all members of the hospital family "owning" the document cannot be overemphasized. "The family that plans together, stays together."

Planning is not entirely a series of definitive and consecutive tasks. There is no set of steps that must always be followed. There will be an occasional shifting of priorities, and directional changes will occur whenever the environment requires it. That is why constant updating is necessary. Planning directions must be made available on a timely basis. Flexibility is encouraged, but you must control flexibility.

Since sound budgeting (see Chapter 15), flows from planning decisions, a master timetable of planning must be created and revised when necessary. For example, Medicare regulations require hospitals to have a three-year capital budget updated annually; without intensive and extensive planning, such a budget would be housed in guesswork. The role of budgeting is increasing in importance each year, and unless it is a part of the planning process, budgeting will fail and the hospital could find itself in fiscal jeopardy.

It is absolutely essential that the future of your hospital should be organized such that the services you provide are not a product of *reaction* to community, medical staff, and dictates of political and cultural change, but rather a result of deliberately planned actions that evolved from the hospital family together with input from the board, administration, medical staff, and the community.

The Role of Strategy in Planning

Your hospital performs strategic planning when you consciously combine the key information available to you (such as service area data, market position, and other environmental issue information) in an *optimum* way to ensure the fulfillment of your stated mission and achievement of board-approved objectives. The key to strategy is *how* you combine your assets. All behavior that is strategic seeks to maximize something, and that is why random behavior can never be strategic. For example, a hospital with strained administrative-medical staff relations may adopt the strategy of involvement: medical staff appointments to the planning committee and even to the board.

Many hospitals appear to have the same insurance mix, a similar medical staff, and many other areas of similarity, and yet one hospital is seen moving forward much better than another. This happens in most communities throughout the country. The key ingredient in strategy and strategic planning is the leadership of the CEO. When the long-range plan is completed, it defines only the orchestra, not the conductor.

We do not intend to leave out the importance of a strong board and well-rounded physician leadership, but that is precisely where the strategy comes in. How many times have we seen a CEO "asleep at the switch?" How many times has it appeared that a particular hospital's board has not moved forward to ensure the maximization of community service? How many times have we seen patient care deteriorate and the CEO coming up with all kinds of reasons and justifications without taking that same creativity and rechanneling it into making corrections and moving forward?

The most important asset of your hospital is people power. An effective board, competent administration, and a well-rounded medical staff certainly should provide the base for assimilating a total management team and professional team, both in direct patient care employees as well as employees in non–patient care departments. You should not overlook volunteers, either. All of these people are the heart of your organization. The hospital that has a good location, adequate parking, a great history, but that does not pay attention to the development of key people and recruitment of key professionals will lose its market position and whatever strategic or competitive advantage that may have once existed.

Developing a comprehensive strategy includes financial areas as well as dealings with areawide hospitals, state health department, the fire marshal, Joint Commission on Accreditation of Hospitals (JCAH), insurance agencies, local political leaders, and others.

Introducing strategy into comprehensive health planning for your hospital is no simple task. According to Peter Drucker, "Management has no choice but to anticipate the future, to attempt to mold it, and to balance short range and long range goals."[2] What we desire for the future will not happen if we just wish hard enough. There are decisions to make and risks to be taken. A classic statement has been provided by Peter Drucker as follows: "Long range planning should prevent managers from uncritically extending present trends into the future, from assuming that today's products, services, markets and technologies will be the products, services, markets, and technologies of tomorrow, and above all, from dedicating their resources and energies to the defense of yesterday."[3] What exists is growing old!

Strategic planning is a logical process that requires analytical thinking. There is very little forecasting in strategic planning because effective CEOs will change their estimated probabilities and assumptions upon which predictions are based. The effective leader makes things happen. Strategic planning does not relate merely to future decisions, but rather to the futurity of present decisions.[4]

The issue is how to "phrase the question." We are not asking what your hospital should be doing tomorrow, but rather, what should you be doing today in order to become ready for an uncertain tomorrow. It is important to choose rationally among the various risks that are part of the various courses of action. It does no good to plunge into uncertainty on the face of guesswork or hunch.

Strategic planning is "a continuous process of making present entrepreneurial (risk-taking) decisions systematically and with the greatest knowledge of their futurity; organizing systematically the effort needed to carry out these decisions; and measuring the results of these decisions against the expectations through organized, systematic feedback."[5]

In our quest to better serve the community, hospitals often add programs but seldom delete programs. It has only been in recent years, with so much duplication of services and the extreme emphasis placed upon cost-containment, that hospitals are beginning to consider deletion of certain services (such as pediatrics, obstetrics, cardiac catheterization).

Your plan should not speak merely of the new things you are going to do and the additional programs you are going to develop and the new markets you are going to serve. Obviously these are important issues, but they should not be the only issues. You may find it better to retrench in one area and expand in another. You need an organized system of change.

Cost-based reimbursement in past years has reduced the motivation to delete services that were duplicated in nearby hospitals. Changes in hospital reimbursement that are now pending will alter much of this and intensify the importance of sound planning. Not all community hospitals will be able to afford to be all things to all people.

When should a hospital delete, expand, or add a particular service? The simplistic answer is that such decisions should reflect the needs of the community. Many hospital emergency departments, for example, do not earn a profit for the hospital. The same may be true in hemodialysis or pediatrics. What your hospital can afford will be a strong determining factor of what service you provide.

There are some services that are essential to general hospitals and would not be likely candidates for deletion. Obviously, the entire medical/surgical inpatient capability of the general acute hospital should remain intact. Many of the surgical subspecialties such as orthopedics need to be a part of most large hospitals. Of course there are exceptions, but the important point is that a study should be made as to which services are candidates for deletion or which should be retained.

As reimbursement restraints emerge, hospitals will become more selective in the expansion of services. If these restraints intensify, marginal services will be dropped. As this continues, mergers and consolidations will occur more and more. Multihospital systems are the wave of the future that has already splashed down. Enter now the conglomerateur, the polycorporate shaker, who will be the new CEO of the future.[6]

FORCES SHAPING PLANNING

External Forces

It is the responsibility of governance in every hospital to determine the programs and services of the hospital. These programs and services are influenced by both external and internal factors. Among the external factors are the following:

- Regulation: Certificate of Need. The most important piece of federal legislation affecting planning was the National Health Planning and Resources Development Act of 1974 (P.L. 93-641). This law set up the mechanism for the creation of HSAs all over the country; hospitals that were contemplating a building program or construction update or purchase of equipment that exceeded $100,000 had to have a certificate of need, and the first step in obtaining such a certificate of need was an approval from the local HSA. This federal initiative gave a great impetus to strategic planning for hospitals. The purpose of this federal legislation was to coordinate the delivery of health care in such a way as to reduce duplication and contain the escalation of health care costs. This law, together with amendments, has forced planning sophistication among our nation's hospitals.

  Unfortunately, in the groundswell to develop short-range projects that would serve the community and satisfy the HSAs created by legislation, there was a bypassing of some major steps that must be taken by hospitals to achieve excellence in planning. (A preparation of a sound mission statement is one.) Maximizing effective patient care may have been aided by P.L. 93-641, but it cannot be done well without the development of a sound mission, formulation of achievable objectives, and assembling the resources necessary for achievement. Even then, there is still more. Involvement and commitment in planning are also necessary, and this is the inner secret of planning for results.

  With the advent of the Reagan administration in 1981, three key potential trends have suddenly emerged: deregulation, increased competition, and changes in reimbursement structure.[7] Levels of federal spending in health care planning will be reduced dramatically. There will be a shift of power to the states in planning, and a large number of federal regulations will be reduced. As this unfolds in the years ahead, the importance of strategic planning will intensify.
- Reimbursement realities. There have been many changes in the manner in which hospitals receive their revenue in the past ten years. Generally the trend has been toward a greater restriction of revenue for hospitals. Cost reimbursement, "cost-plus" reimbursement, prospective reimbursement, state rate review committees, among others, have all undergone change, and the outlook is for even more severe revenue restriction in health care in the years ahead.
- Competition. Sophistication in planning and the preparation of strategic plans by hospitals often results in increasing competitiveness of health care facilities within the community. There have been arguments that competition increases the cost of health care delivery,

that instead there should be sharing of information and services, and that there should be communication in order to avoid duplication of services. On the other hand, warnings have come to the forefront that suggest that competition will have a positive effect on health care costs among the better-run hospitals. Only the more competitive hospitals will survive.

Richard L. Johnson speaks of the upcoming radical changes that will occur in our nation's health care delivery system as the public, labor, management, and government force our system to enter the mainstream of American life, where he feels that the ability to successfully compete in a free marketplace will determine the winners and losers.[8] There will be great emphasis on improving productivity and pricing services on marginal cost concepts and pushing hospital management practices into economic competition. He points out that parts of P.L. 93-641 have built-in barriers to provide for effective competition, as three of the ten guidelines used in evaluating a hospital's application for certificate of need refer to cooperative planning.

According to the guidelines, a hospital is expected to develop its plan and share the information with the other institutions in the same area and secure their cooperation. Therefore, the sharing of price and cost information between institutions is not only not penalized but is considered a desirable activity. In other industries the activity could be illegal, since it may be regarded as collusion or restraint of trade. There has been much discussion of this in the hospital literature in regard to directions that may be taken in the future by the Department of Justice.

The Health Planning and Resources Development Amendments of 1979 dictated changes in the way the certificate-of-need process takes place. In addition, the amendments will encourage more competition, and proposed services that increase such competition in community health care are most likely to be approved.[9] It will behoove hospitals to stress the competitive aspects of their proposals in certificate-of-need applications.

Some other areas provided for in the 1979 amendments include the fact that new services with an expected annual operating cost exceeding $75,000 will come under the jurisdiction of the HSA; this provision could limit the expansion of services and actually create an anticompetitive bias towards hospitals that may be already performing the service regardless of how well they are doing it. The minimum dollar amount for construction or purchase of equipment requiring a certificate of need has been increased to $150,000 from $100,000. In addition, the HSAs are required to provide hospitals with technical assistance in preparing their certificate-of-need applications. That same kind of technical assistance will be helpful to hospitals in the data phase of their planning process. Many of these issues will change dramatically as the federal initiative in planning subsides. The HSAs that survive from state funding or other funding will have changed roles, and hospitals will need to be able to adapt to all these external factors that bear upon their planning.

Alfred Kahn, federal inflation fighter, spoke at the National Journal's health policy conference in Washington, DC and noted that there are several procompetition consumer choice proposals in Congress. He proposed that the system be as self-regulating as possible, in a way that a competitive market is self-regulating.[10]

Some further issues on the role of competition in health care have been noted by Columbia University economist, Eli Ginsberg, Ph.D., who argued that competition already exists, and that advocates of the so-called pro-competition plans are too quick to reject regulatory attempts to control costs.[11]

Dr. Saudek reported that the competitive approach to controlling the costs is a necessary alternative to regulation. He believes that competition does not exist and that it will not until consumers have more at stake financially when they select a health care plan. He also said that "hospitals compete for patients, but never on a price basis . . . he concluded that the real question is whether or not it could ever exist."[12]

The attention of the federal government on the role of competition in health care was described by Donald W. Moran:

> If we can restore some confidence that the amount of money that we are spending on health care is the result of conscious choices made in the face of rational incentives, it simply does not matter how much national income the American people choose to spend on health care. Unlike the quasi-public-utility model on which current federal regulatory efforts are based, pro-competition seeks to tear down existing barriers to the promotion of ever-greater quality medical care at reasonable costs.[13]

- Strategies in dealing with HSAs and state health departments. Actions of federal, state, and local governments will continue to influence the development of hospital services and programs. There are many strategies available to health care institutions in dealing with the HSAs and state health departments in order to obtain a certificate of need. This process requires the hospital to perform, in many instances, a comprehensive market analysis. Some of the criteria used by HSAs to evaluate proposals submitted to them for a certificate of need are demonstrated community need, ability to staff and operate, physical design, quality of care, financial issues, economic issues, organizational issues, and consumer involvement and support, including the support of projects by adjacent community hospitals.

- Public pressure. Every hospital must attempt to become a solid part of the community. This will help raise money with local bankers, facilitate a fund drive for capital formation, and facilitate recruitment of physicians, paramedical professionals, and others. Community support is a very important external source that will help shape the planning of your hospital.

  For example, your hospital has an emergency department for which the local community feels the wait to receive care is generally too long or the prices of services are excessive or the professional conduct of nurses, physicians, and other persons in the emergency department is not satisfactory. Patients will seek other alternatives if other alternatives are or become available. The strategic plan for your hospital should ensure that these kinds of major problems do not occur in your inpatient care, your outpatient care, or in any other facet of the hospital that deals with patients, visitors, and the general public.

- Technology and resources. Included here are many external areas that will affect your planning process. There have been many examples of hospitals that were ready to update their physical facility, but when they went into the capital market they found the interest rates, even for tax-exempt bonds, to be well over 10 percent. While the interest rates in the bond market are not controllable by the hospital, there are still many strategies available that your hospital can employ to obtain the best possible interest rate for capital formation. In working with underwriters a great deal of homework must be done in order that a sound picture of your hospital is brought forth. This will have some potential influence on the bond rating of your hospital. Key board members and major members of the medical staff need to lend their support in special meetings that will have to be held during the process of moving toward obtaining tax-exempt bond financing.

  Another example is energy. As the cost and the availability of energy create challenges for your hospital, you will need to prepare special strategies and special alternative approaches to minimize the negative effects. In addition, there are many decisions a hospital needs to make regarding automation, such as computerization of many areas related to the business side of the hospital as well as the patient care areas. If your hospital is not up-to-date with computerization in areas other than office procedures, such as CT scanning, it will be at a disadvantage.

- Health maintenance organizations (HMOs). Even though we may see less financial support from the government in HMOs, there is still going to be a long-run trend in the increasing utilization and power of HMOs. Partly because of the pressures from their medical staffs as well as other reasons, there have been a great many hospitals that have not looked very favorably toward the affiliation with HMOs. There are many arguments that they can allegedly reduce the cost of health care, yet the question is raised whether consumers will be satisfied not having the patient-physician relationship to which so many of us have been accustomed.

  One major strategy available to many hospitals, rather than ignore or fight HMOs, is to establish relationships with them. Such relationships can be quite extensive or of a more general nature. You might even find an advantage in working with one or two other hospitals in your community to establish an HMO. You should be in control of your destiny rather than have these external factors begin to control you. Only by establishing a sound planning process can you face the issues of HMOs effectively.
- Demographics: ethnic, education, age, migration/immigration, income levels. All of these affect utilization and the planning process at your hospital. These areas are covered in Chapter 5.

This has been a discussion of the external factors that affect hospital governance in the development of hospital services and programs. Most of these are at least partly beyond the control of the hospital. However, among the internal factors there is some degree of control available to the health care facility. Among these would be the nature, type, and age of the medical staff, ability to staff the hospital, financial factors, as well as the quality of management. This entire area will be discussed in detail in Chapter 5.

National, State, and Local Objectives

Stemming from the federal initiative, we have seen the formulation of objectives (generally referred to as goals) at the federal, state, and local levels. P.L. 93-641, as we have previously mentioned, had as a major objective the containment of health care costs. Other objectives of this law were to develop a national health policy, augment state and regional health planning, and authorize financial assistance for the development of resources to further the national health policy. According to Paul Ward, president of the California Hospital Association, "P.L. 93-641 is a negative, costly, destructive process that is built upon misleading statements of intent and fallacious assumptions. The basic problem is that health planning is not a planning but a regulatory process. Planning began after World War II as a way of bringing services to people; now it has become a regulatory means of attempting to keep services from people."[14] As a direct result of this law, government agencies at the local, state, and national levels have prepared sets of health goals and guidelines for achievement.

We will now present a summary of the goals at each level and describe how they are interrelated.

National Guidelines

Guidelines at the national level are formulated for two reasons: to establish and coordinate national health policy and to assist regional HSAs in developing their regional health systems plans (HSPs). They are prepared in two parts. The first part that was issued in 1978 specifies standards to be applied in planning the supply, distribution, and organization of health resources. For example, these standards may apply to hospital beds, facilities for open-heart surgery, CT scanners, cardiac catheterization, radiation therapy, and end-stage renal disease programs. The second section of the national guidelines is in the proposal stage. This contains only one set of goals that addresses institutional and personal resources and systems of care such as access to care, shared services, and primary care, and another set of goals pertaining to disease prevention, health promotion, and health status outcomes (such as accident prevention, childhood diseases, and mortality rates). Periodically all the national goals and standards will be revised, and additional ones presented. Such information becomes a key part of the environmental analysis of every hospital and can serve as major information for the determination of objectives for your hospital. The same is true for the state and regional guidelines.

State Guidelines

The preparation of a State Health Plan (SHP) is required by both P.L. 93-641 and laws enacted by a particular state. For example, in Michigan there is the Michigan Health Planning and Resources Development Act of 1978. The proposed Michigan SHP was written by the Statewide Health Coordinating Council (SHCC) with the assistance of the Office of Health and Medical Affairs (OHMA). This model is not unique to Michigan but exists in many states, although not all states have yet adopted a final plan. The SHP is required to be composed of the regional HSP of the HSAs within the state, revised to achieve statewide coordination or to deal more effectively with statewide needs. Since the individual SHPs are already consistent with the National Health Planning Guidelines, the regional HSP will also reflect these goals. The SHP is only a planning guideline document to be used as a resource in the creation of statewide health policy.

Most of the goals in a typical SHP are included in the regional HSP, although probably in less ambitious terms. In the State of Michigan we can present to you the following example:

> The 1980–84 Preliminary State Health Plan will be acted upon by the Statewide Health Coordinating Council (S.H.C.C.). The S.H.C.C. State Health Plan Development Committee, although acting without a quorum, has recommended to the S.H.C.C. that the State Health Plan include:
>
> 1. A goal of achieving an 800-day per thousand population medical/surgical patient day use rate for acute care hospitals in this state, the result of which would be the identification of approximately 7,000 more "excess beds" in Michigan hospitals.
> 2. A reduction from 4.26 to 3.87 average length of stay for obstetric bed needs planning.
> 3. The requirement that hospitals annually report, for the future 5-year period, all proposed capital expenditures which will exceed $1 million or change the services or bed supply of the institution."[15]

Information from the SHP of your state, as part of your environmental analysis, constitutes the basis for objectives to be prepared! Some of the examples of objectives that should be considered are to target reductions, if appropriate, in the average length of stay for various services such as pediatrics, obstetrics, medical/surgical patients, and so forth.

Another example is that if, in a given state, the hospital utilization rate was 1,400 days per 1,000 patient population, one of the ways for individual hospitals to reduce this would be to expand their program of ambulatory surgery.

Local Guidelines

Let us examine the regional goals of local HSAs. P.L. 93-641 requires that the HSPs of each HSA take into account and be consistent with national guidelines, although recent amendments soften this to ensure that local plans meet local needs. At the same time, these HSAs must take into account the needs, resources, and priorities of their areas and confront important local problems not addressed in the national guidelines.

We will now develop an example that may serve to clarify this. In the greater Detroit area, the local HSA is the Comprehensive Health Planning Council of Southeastern Michigan (CHPC-SEM). The regional goals (in this book we are treating goals and objectives as synonyms), of CHPC-SEM are categorized into three levels of priority. The top level is categorized as Category 1. These goals address problems of significant importance and amenability to local solution. For this level, goals, objectives, and recommended actions are identified. (In this framework goals are defined as the highest obtainable standards, while objectives represent expected achievement.) Category II goals identify issues of lesser importance for which solid objectives can be formulated. Category III, "community concerns," are nonquantifiable problems felt by CHPC-SEM to require recognition. Thus the HSP contains goals addressing almost all of the problems for which national guidelines were issued back in 1978 and for many of the problems addressed in the currently proposed set.

HSAs have limited authority to achieve their goals, and achievement is generally done through the issuance of a certificate of need and an appropriateness review of new and existing programs and services that are presented to HSA. The certificate-of-need process is the vehicle by which HSAs can have an impact on shaping the health care system. HSAs are encouraged by the Department of Health and Human Services to work with providers, insurers, and federal, state, and community agencies to achieve their goals. The efforts of HSAs to move toward their goals are monitored, although they may not be able to attain all of them since such attainment is a complex process involving the entire health care provider system on a local basis.

There is no question that hospitals should look to the HSP that affects their service area as a partial basis for some of their formulation of objectives. For example, the HSA plan may have a target of 20 percent of all surgery to be performed on an ambulatory basis by a certain year. If a particular hospital has no formal program of ambulatory surgery, or perhaps a program with only 5 percent or 10 percent, realistic objectives should be formulated by the planning committee. There are many strategies that will need to be developed to achieve a certain level of ambulatory surgery, and cooperation between and among administration and medical staff will be of obvious importance.

If HSAs continue to survive, and it is unlikely that many of them will, it is possible that we will see down the road an evaluation by an HSA of hospitals that present a request for certificate of need, and a close examination of how that hospital meets the objectives in its HSP. An obvious example of what an HSA may do would be that if a hospital were going to replace 50 of its inpatient beds because of code violations, the HSA may examine such issues as the level of ambulatory surgery and the average length of stay in each of their services and determine that only 20 or 30 (or some other number) of those 50 beds should be replaced.

There has been, is now, and will continue to be major conflicts between some hospitals and their HSA in their certificate-of-need negotiations.

> HSAs must respond not only to federal planning criteria, but also to a variety of opinions from a wide range of interest groups. In making conclusions, HSAs must strike a balance among diverse viewpoints, so their planning and policy documents frequently reflect a consensus of the conventional, or at least acceptable, wisdom. Hospital planning, however, is a private enterprise. Although the final plan document often is made public, the debates and negotiations among various groups within the hospital during the planning process are conducted in relative privacy . . . from these differences between HSAs and hospitals emerge dramatic differences in the results of their planning efforts.
>
> Hospitals, at their best, conduct sound corporate planning. They perceive their future strength in terms of their response to community needs through diversification of services and, more recently, through outreach and satellite programs. In pursuing their goals, they have continuity of organizational leadership combined with their economic and political strength as employers of large numbers of people. In contrast, HSAs search for opportunity to reduce inpatient costs.[16]

Pierce has offered some strategies for hospitals in responding to the challenges of HSAs and suggests that hospitals develop a sound corporate plan. He suggests that hospital officials begin negotiating early for their certificate of need applications and involve the HSA staff members and committee members early in the planning of proposed new programs; he also suggests that hospital officials expand their roles on HSA committees, and that each hospital should make a strong effort, through education, to teach HSA staff, board, and committee members about the dynamics of hospital operations. This is a key part of strategic planning, and the CEO, as conductor of the orchestra, makes these kinds of things happen.

Among the more important issues to recognize is that hospitals can and must develop their challenges to the HSA through sound strategic planning with their administration, board, and medical staffs, but at the same time it must be recognized that planning has a totally different orientation for hospitals than for HSAs and that there will never likely be an integration of where each is coming from.

In a speech given in Washington in early 1980, Symond Gottleib predicted defeat of the National Health Planning and Resources Development Act of 1974 when it comes up for renewal in 1982. The speech, given to members of the American Hospital Association, expressed his views that there tends to be a lack of consistent local planning administration, public support, and performance evaluation in local health planning. Gottleib stated that

> HSAs lack credibility, are not perceived as competent, not handling tough issues objectively, have not established a general direction of health services development, and are not active catalysts in bringing about needed change in the health care system . . . . I see in the future, after HSAs are emasculated . . . a return to health planning, as an organized process of thinking before action is taken.[17]

WHERE ARE WE NOW?

In the past few years there has been an enormous maturing of hospitals regarding their planning process. Planning staffs have grown from an administrative assistant performing statistical analysis to much larger departments of planning headed by a department head reporting to the CEO, or in many cases, an assistant administrator or vice-president for the planning function has emerged. The combination of greater expectations of health care on the part of the community served by hospitals and the reduced financial resources with which to serve the documented needs of the community has resulted in a high priority being given to the planning process, which is dictated by hospital governance and followed through by competent administration! "Once it was sufficient for a hospital to have a building committee. Today the hospital needs a committee that can assess its environment, its internal strengths and weaknesses, and the role of the hospital as an entity should fill within its community."[18]

Twenty years ago there were very few planning committees in hospitals. Nearly ten years ago there were long-range planning committees in approximately 77 percent of our nation's hospitals.[19] Today there is hardly a successful hospital without a viable planning committee.

Without an effective framework for planning, however, the benefits will be limited. The purpose of the planning process is not to come up with facilities, construction priorities, and new programs. The primary purpose of this process is to determine who we are and what we are about, and to do this by assimilating key members of the board, the administration, and the medical staff, with appropriate community input, to work through the planning process together as a group, so that, as the results of planning pour forth, there is a commitment of ownership on the part of the entire hospital family! We have mentioned previously the importance of the hospital "owning" the document, and it will continue to be mentioned. Involvement is the secret.

Input and deliberations from other board committees, such as the finance committee and quality assurance committee, among others, as well as administrative committees and the executive committee of the medical staff, will be necessary on a continuing basis.

The full process of planning begins with plan development and moves to program development, to financial factors related to program development, to implementation, and then to evaluation; the cycle continues with feedback into the planning process as we have presented it. The cycle will continue because planning never ends.

The planning process will have to be integrated with your hospital's organizational structure in order to determine the most appropriate framework for establishing and continuing an ongoing process. Even before a planning committee is formed, it is necessary for your hospital to determine who should have input to the planning process. The significant environmental factors and the input process should be determined.

The pressure for formation of a planning committee in a hospital goes back to 1970 with the announcement of standards from the JCAH. It was recommended that a hospital appoint a separate planning body or a committee to do the hospital planning. The formation of a planning committee is a major step. Unless its agenda has sound direction and addresses itself to major in-depth planning issues such as who we are and what we are about, the output will be of little value.

There must be a realistic consideration of the needs of a community by the planning committee, or the members will not feel any sense of identity with other health care institutions and providers that are a part of the process, too. If it is not done right, members will become frustrated because the process takes so long or because they have so little to show for their efforts. Members will lose confidence and attendance will diminish.

Sometimes we see a hospital with good momentum in developing programs to meet community needs; however, when the planning committee is appointed and it starts concentrating on philosophical issues, it appears that the momentum has been lost, when actually the planning process is now beginning rather than concluding.

> A (planning) committee can function effectively if it can lift itself out of the goal-setting syndrome and if it defines its role clearly and realistically in terms of the new and dynamic relationships that are developing between the hospital and its environment. Environmental analysis and planning provide a clear-cut framework for the committee to define its role within the institution and for it to outline appropriate and specific tasks for itself within that role.[20]

The primary function of the planning committee is to serve as an extension of the board, whereby the planning process is guided by involving the major members of the entire hospital family and community; in addition, the planning committee has a very important educational role. It has a major function of communication and

> may also be able to serve as the support system for change. Any change is a wrench, particularly if the changes are of a deep and profound nature, as in health care. These changes are causing a terrible dislocation. Although some committees find governing bodies resistant to change, more find that the major source of resistance is the medical staff, many of whom are independent professionals and still behave as if the hospital were their workshop.[21]

ORGANIZING THE PLANNING FUNCTION

The planning committee should be designated by the board and chaired by a member of the board of trustees as a committee of the board. The committee chairperson should be carefully chosen by the chairperson of the board. The composition of the committee should include two or three additional members from the board of trustees, significant representation from the medical staff (both in number and in the choices made), the CEO, one or more other key members of hospital administration including expertise in planning, and community representation. This latter category could include a representative from the local visiting nursing association, a neighborhood block club president or other civic board officer, and anyone else that can provide a well-rounded community flavor.

There is no cookbook set of guidelines on how to make these choices. For example, a hospital that selects for its medical staff representation four hospital-based physicians and no members from the private practice physicians may find itself with a great deal of criticism right from the start. Appointing members from private practice who are too busy or not sufficiently interested to attend the meetings will result in a different set of problems. Balance is the key; physicians who are motivated and who represent the medical staff generally by being in private practice are often appointed with the greatest degree of success.

The committee should be large enough to have good input and small enough to get things done. There is no magic number, and an optimum size should be the objective. In many hospitals the average size is 9 to 12 members.

Additional involvement can be accomplished by having subcommittees appointed by the planning committee. Rotation of membership on the planning subcommittees is effective, but there should be limited rotation on the planning committee itself in order to provide continuity. It goes without saying that the committee must have adequate staff support in order to do all the homework that will be necessary between meetings.

Monthly meetings of one to two hours are commonly held. At certain times in the planning process a full day retreat may be deemed necessary. Meetings held in the morning when people are fresh and the medical staff more readily available are more profitable. Three o'clock meetings will frequently lose the private practitioners, since in many instances this is in the middle of their office schedule. These are issues that the committee itself can easily address. The planning committee should be given a specific written charge by the governing board that will outline the directions of their responsibility and their authority.

An important element in the planning process is for the hospital to have on board the person who is going to direct the planning activity for the hospital before the planning process starts. It is not wise judgment to have the planning committee prepare the plan and then the CEO hire the person to follow up the plan after it has been prepared. Regardless of the title for the hospital planner (such as vice-president for planning), the role of that function should be identified as being very important to the overall planning process, both in developing the process and in ensuring that it is being carried out.

SUMMARY

In conclusion, every hospital must make a major decision regarding how committed it will be to the planning process. It cannot be done part way and be effective. If we are really committed to quality patient care, then we are of necessity committed to the rigor of the planning process. Long-run maximization of quality patient care cannot be assured without successful planning all along the way. The survival of your hospital is at stake.

NOTES

1. Richard L. Johnson, "The 1980s: The Rise of HMOs and Marketplace Competition," *Hospital Progress,* June 1979, pp. 38–43.

2. Peter F. Drucker, *Management* (New York: Harper & Row, 1974), p. 121.

3. Ibid., p. 122.

4. Ibid., p. 124.

5. Ibid., p. 125.

6. Montague Brown, "The Administrator as Master Strategist," Annual Convocation of the American Academy of Medical Administrators, Las Vegas, Oct. 6, 1981.

7. According to Donald W. Moran, "Under an effective regulatory regime, overbuilding and overuse are punished by being reimbursed at only 85% of one's cost; under price competition on the basis of total medical service delivery via planned premiums, the result of excess is absolute insolvency." *Hospitals,* Feb. 16, 1981, p. 48.

8. Richard L. Johnson, "HMOs and Marketplace Competition," *Hospital Progress,* July 1979, pp. 38–43. See also his article entitled "The Caterpillar and the Butterfly: Despite Regulations, the System Thrives," *Hospital Progress,* April 1980, pp. 54–61.

9. Esther Kuntz, "Public Law 96-79 Changes C.O.N. Processes," *Modern Health Care,* Nov. 1979, p. 50.

10. *Hospital Week,* June 20, 1980, p. 2.

11. Ibid., p. 2.

12. Ibid., p. 3.

13. *Hospitals,* Feb. 16, 1981, p. 38.

14. *CHA News,* Nov. 7, 1980, p. 1.

15. Michigan Hospital Association, *Monday Report,* March 24, 1980, p. 1.

16. J. Pierce and F. Charles, "H.S.A., Hospital Planning: Arena of Conflict Offers Room for Cooperation," *Hospitals,* March 16, 1980, pp. 63–64.

17. Symond Gottleib, speech delivered to American Hospital Association, Washington, DC, 1980.

18. James Webber and Marsha A. Dula, "Effective Planning Committees for Hospitals," *Harvard Business Review,* May–June 1974, p. 51.

19. Martin S. Perlin, "Current Practices in Long Range Planning," *Hospitals,* Sept. 1, 1972, p. 62.

20. Webber, "Effective Planning Committees," p. 54.

21. Ibid., p. 58.

Chapter 5

How to Prepare a Long-Range Master Plan

MISSION STATEMENT

The foundation upon which all planning is built is the mission statement of your hospital. There is no way to effectively develop community service programs without really knowing who you are and what you are about.

A comprehensive mission statement tells you what you believe, gives you consistency of purpose, and becomes the framework for all your hospital policy formulation. It is your source of direction, your reason for being, and it acknowledges all your community relationships:

You need to know where you have been, where you are now, agreed upon, and in writing.

Some of the questions you must consider include:

- What do we believe about us? (What are our ideals?)
- What should we believe in?
- Why are we here?
- Why should we be here?
- What are we now?
- What do we wish to become?
- Who are we serving?
- Who should we serve?
- Where are we headed?
- Where should we be headed?
- What services do we offer?
- What services should we offer? When? Why?

The mission or purpose of an organization is ongoing and never-ending. It is something for which you constantly strive, and it will never be achieved completely. For a business firm it might be to produce and sell the highest quality product or service possible at the lowest cost consistent with making a profit for the owners. For an educational institution it might often be expressed as contributing to the formation, education, and growth of mature citizens such as to enhance the quality of life relevant to human needs. For a health care facility it might be to provide the highest possible patient care consistent with the ability of payers to underwrite the cost.

The mission is a credo and a statement of the values to which you are committed. It is the philosophy particular tc the organization that attracts individuals and that they, in turn, seek to mirror in their personal lives and actions. Business firms often express such credos in terms of their commitments. They are committed to their employees, their customers, the general population, the law, and so forth. Volunteer organizations, including religious, youth, and welfare groups in society, prosper depending upon their ability to project their beliefs to the public and to gain sufficient monetary and personal support to survive.

Synonyms for a mission statement include:

- credo
- philosophy
- role
- organizational purpose
- statement of ideals
- statement of values
- statement of beliefs

In this book, we are treating all these as part of a single statement of mission. Some hospitals separate them, and one of the schemes is to develop a separate:

- philosophy (fundamental beliefs)
- mission (fundamental purposes)
- role (fundamental directions)

In Exhibit 5-1 we have shown both approaches and how to go from one to the other. Our reason for suggesting to our readers the combined approach is that no matter how carefully you define the terms and no matter how clearly a long list of examples is presented, it is often difficult to separate and classify all the elements into different categories. Some of the role issues get mixed in with mission issues and vice versa. This doesn't mean it's wrong to separate, only that it is more useful to combine.

Exhibit 5-1 A Checklist for the Preparation of Your Mission Statement

COMPREHENSIVE MISSION STATEMENT	*Philosophy*	*Theological*	1. Belief in God, Judeo/Christian ethics. 2. Belief in the Catholic Church, other denominations. a. The church as a healing mission. 3. Belief in Christ's active love for all persons, including the needy, suffering, lonely, powerless and the oppressed.
		General	4. Reverence for life; belief in the patient's right to care when he is ill, and the right to die in dignity and peace. 5. Philosophy on abortions, sterilization, euthanasia. 6. Beliefs regarding the hospital's dedication to preserving the value, dignity, and quality of life of all patients served without regard to race, religion, sex, age, creed, or ability to pay.
	Mission		7. Provide services that enhance the dignity and quality of life of all patients and other persons served by the hospital (such as doctors, employees, visitors) a. Commitment to employees could include providing fair wages, hours, and working conditions; dedicated personnel will be sought in all new hires; (commitment to affirmative action?); their professional growth will be provided for by training and education programs, proper placement policies, promotion from within whenever possible, and the sound exercise of participate management at all levels of administrative organization. b. Commitment to the medical staff—bringing in highly qualified members; open dialogue and communication—fostering true teamwork with medical staff, board, and administration; full recognition of their needs and values. 8. Will educational programs be offered (such as residency training, patient education, and employee professional development)? 9. Will active outreach be conducted to serve the underserved, as a major thrust of the hospital? 10. Will the entire range of patient care be targeted to a specific patient grouping (such as children, adult psychiatry)? 11. Degree of commitment to cost-containment in the delivery of health care? To preventive care? To coordinated areawide planning? To sharing services and information with other health care providers in the area? To alternative methods of health care delivery? 12. To bring about the healing work of Christ in the community served. 13. To providing quality health care at the highest level consistent with the limits of the hospital's human, technological, and financial resources.

Exhibit 5-1 continued

	Role	14. What extent of programs in primary, secondary, and/or tertiary care will be provided? 15. Will the hospital seek to determine if there are any gaps in the provision of community health care? If there are, will programs be studied for possible implementation? 16. Degree of commitment to serve the "downtown" area, "inner-city"? 17. Special programs of outreach; the elderly, sickle cell testing; ambulatory care satellites in ghetto areas. 18. Will the hospital establish a referral network for patients requiring services they do not have? 19. Determine research role and type, such as clinical; will ties be established or maintained with a medical school and how closely and why? 20. Is your hospital a community health resource, concentrating on the provisions for health promotion and health maintenance aspects through neighborhood health screening, child health screening and immunization, and categorical health teaching programs (e.g., hypertension, diabetes)? The programs offered should be proven as to meeting the needs of the target population, through research based methodology.

In Exhibit 5-1 a checklist of 20 areas is presented. These were taken from actual hospital mission statements from around the country. The more comprehensive your mission statement is, the stronger will be the basis for the objectives you will be formulating. This doesn't mean that your mission should be long; it means it should be crisp, integrated, and complete. Not all 20 items from Exhibit 5-1 need be included, and perhaps others should be in it. It is merely a guideline for you, a way to find something you may have left out and wanted in.

The mission statement is the most essential element in the planning process.

> It is suggested that the mission statement for small and rural hospitals should define the hospital's role or responsibility in advocating and coordinating access for its service area population to all necessary health care, regardless of the geographic location of that care. In addition, it is further suggested that the mission statement should define the upper levels of care to be rendered by that institution.[1]

It is very important that there be a good deal of involvement in the preparation of the mission statement. Main direction may come from the board-approved planning committee, but it is also necessary to involve all members of the board, medical staff leaders, administration, the sponsors (depending upon the kind of hospital), and other members of the hospital family, as appropriate.

Sometimes a good place to start in developing a mission statement is to examine the bylaws and/or articles of incorporation. The first draft may seem to come easy, but be prepared to expect a large number of revisions. There will not be agreement by all members of the hospital family as to the various elements of the mission statement. If agreement comes too easily, it may indicate that not enough dialogue went into the discussion. It is just as important for the hospital family to own the mission statement as it is that they own and feel committed to the entire planning process and to the written plan after it is developed.

The mission statement is not a secret document. It should be placed in many of the major documents of your hospital, such as the annual report of services and patient information brochures, among others. The public should know about it.

The reason it is so important to have all the hospital family aware on a regular basis of your mission is because it highlights the ideals that to some measure become the reason that many of your members stay with you over the coming years. All should be committed to the ideals presented in the mission statement.

One important function of a mission statement is to fly the flag and to keep up the morale of the troops, to be the banner waving over the dust and smoke of the day-to-day battles, to render maximum community care under severely curtailed resources, and to be a beacon to all who belong with you. Motivation is a key word that you want to remember in referring to the mission statement. As you are motivated by similar ideals, you will be a greater part of the team in achieving your objectives in the months and years ahead. You should be proud to wave the flag to outsiders. Your mission is something you wave to others, saying with pride: "Here is what we stand for, here is what we believe in, here is where we are going! Do you share these beliefs, these ideals, these dreams? If so, you might wish to join us; you might wish to join our medical staff, or to become a volunteer, or an employee. You may choose us for your patient care. You might even support us financially. Of course, if you do not share these values, then it is best that you know this now, so as not to be surprised later."

Paramount in your understanding of mission statements should be the organizational principle that structure flows from purpose, function follows form. Before one can begin to be effectively active, there has to be a clear understanding of and commitment to the purpose of the organization and to the subunit within the organization to which one belongs. When the purpose is lost sight of, the door is opened to counterproductive effort. But with a well-stated mission in hand, decisions about operational objectives can be dispassionately made.

In addition to being broad enough to cover the types of programs to be conducted under the aegis of the hospital, a useful mission statement must also be narrow enough to distinguish one hospital from another so that people both inside and outside can choose the particular one with which they wish to align themselves.

It should be noted, however, that not everyone supports a high emphasis on the mission statement of an organization. Richard Chaite throws a caution and suggests that mission statements are not so much valueless as overvalued, that they should not be discarded, only deemphasized.[2] He feels that many mission statements are similar among colleges and universities and makes a plea for distinctiveness, suggesting that there is a quality far more important than uniqueness, that a college need not be different to be distinctive, only better. He concludes by mentioning that the best way to survive, even flourish, may be to worry a little less about mission statements and a little more about actions. While the two are related, we have overworked the former, perhaps because it is not as easy to attend to the latter.

Our definition of a comprehensive mission statement includes all of the following:

1. A determination of your hospital's fundamental beliefs; this enables you to confront all moral and ethical issues you face in the health care field. These beliefs seldom, if ever, change. For example, if a new federal law were passed that required abortions in all hospitals, we would find Roman Catholic hospitals in the political arena and in the courts, and a significant power struggle would emerge. The reason for this is the basic philosophy of Roman Catholic hospitals regarding abortion.
2. A specific statement of purpose, your hospital's *raison d'être*.
3. The specific function of the hospital in providing health care. Based on the services and programs your hospital offers, you can differentiate your role from the role of other hospitals.
4. The level and scope of emphasis of services to be provided (as well as services to be excluded).
5. Acknowledgment of your relationship with your community, other local providers, federal, state, and local governments, regulatory agencies, and health departments, among others.

Appendix 5-A includes sample mission statements of various hospital departments.

THE ORGANIZATION OF THE WRITTEN PLAN FOR YOUR HOSPITAL

There is an old adage that states: "If you do not know where you are going, any road will get you there." We need a plan for planning. Since part of our goal is to produce a written plan, let us describe now what goes into the plan.

There are many ways to organize the contents of the written plan. We will provide for you a specific model that will work for any size hospital. It is up to you to tailor information we present to fit your particular circumstances.

Our attempt here will be to present an outline for planning that will not change regardless of whether there is a large amount of government regulation in planning or a small amount. The key steps that we will describe must still be followed. Only the external environmental factors will be impacted; strategic planning for any health care organization must relate to reality and work through the maze regardless of what the particular restraints or challenges are.

The general concepts of planning for a well-known hospital with a large teaching program and over 1,000 beds is not significantly different nor more important in any way than the planning for a small 70-bed rural hospital with limited medical staff and no teaching program of a formal nature. "It is apparent that individual small and/or rural hospitals which include more than half of the hospitals in the United States may not survive in their present role, location, or service configuration, despite their importance to their communities, unless planning is immediately adopted as a major management function."[3]

Most of the examples we will use will be from the larger hospital, so that if we describe, for example, service area population information with a large number of zip codes, the principles will apply to the small rural hospital, but complexity of data gathering for the smaller hospital will be much less. Our planning model also applies to specialty hospitals, such as children's hospitals or psychiatric hospitals. The model will also apply to general community hospitals, as well as to large tertiary centers connected with medical schools.

From time to time, specific strategies in making these differentiations will be presented when we feel that they would be useful for you.

A Typical Outline for Your Hospital's Plan:

I. General Introduction to Your Hospital
II. Comprehensive Mission Statement
III. Environmental Assessment

IV. Data Determination and Assessment
    A. Service Area Population
    B. Utilization Trends at Your Hospital
    C. Medical Staff Analysis
    D. Demographics
    E. Health Services Inventory
    F. Financial Analysis
V. Issues and Problems
    A. Priorities
VI. Overall Hospital Annual Objectives (See Chapter 6)

Let us now develop this outline in some detail.

General Introduction to Your Hospital

This section should present a description of your hospital and will include such significant information as: Where is it? When did it start and by whom? Progress? What services are offered? Financial status? It is a basic overview of your hospital, short and concise, including number of employees, medical staff, volunteers, what residencies you have (if any), medical education issues, condition of physical facilities.

Comprehensive Mission Statement (Previously covered).

Environmental Assessment

A general environmental assessment of your hospital should be completed. We will now briefly describe how you should develop an overall statement of your hospital environment in relation to national issues. The American Hospital Association prepared such an assessment in 1979; it is very well done and can be used as a base for your own revisions, to come up with what you feel are the main areas in an overall environmental assessment.[4]

A description and some assumptions will be needed about the composition of the hospital industry and its structure and the role of financing, including where you might be headed in rate review or prospective reimbursement. What will happen to regulations, new legislation, law suits? What about human resource development and patient services?

These are major issues in hospital organization that need to be looked at. We need to state our feelings about what is happening to the liability of governing boards. Will it become increasingly difficult to obtain trustees because of liability and other pressures? What impact will this have upon the hospital if it is true?

What about multihospital arrangements, and how will this affect the traditional form of hospital governance? Will we have a surplus of physicians in the next 10 years, or will we merely have an excess of physicians in suburbia?

The long-run survival of professional standard review organizations is in doubt; what effect will this have on the hospital's ability to practice effective utilization review? There will be many changes in the relationships among health care professions, and this will require hospitals to reexamine their organizational structures and lines of accountability. Will there be greater or lesser conflict within the hospital in the physician–administrative arena?

The written statement of your environmental analysis should cover a time period of at least five years, and some hospitals have even attempted to do this on a ten-year basis. The key to this of course is that the longer the timeframe the more difficult it is to be assured that we have a correct statement. We have more confidence in a five-year projection than in a ten-year projection. There are some macroenvironment areas that can be considered in long-range planning.[5]

Data Determination and Assessment

The data in support of this section belongs in a separate appendix, but it is important to summarize the highlights in an organized manner. Some of the areas to include are whether or not you are in an "underserved" area and/or in a manpower shortage area under federal designation: demographic service area information. The issues here should be summarized into external (those that you cannot change) and internal (those that are under the control of the hospital).

The purpose here is to lay out the environment in order to establish the base to draw forth the issues and problems in the next section.

In order to prepare a description of the environment of your hospital, there are six major areas that will be included for analysis. These are service area populations, utilization trends, medical staff analysis, demographics, health services inventory, and financial issues. Such data are very important in order to conduct community-based planning. Your hospital must have an understanding of the health needs and problems of the population that you serve, as well as an understanding of the overall utilization of the entire spectrum of health care resources available to meet the needs of your service population.

Service Area Population. You must be sensitive to confirmed community need while attempting to develop overall strategies for your growth and for the development and organization of your programs, services, manpower, and resources. You start the analysis of your service area population by determining the overall demand in a region, such as in your county or in your health systems area. After the overall population served has been determined, you must specifically focus upon the community that you serve. A patient origin study can be performed by your hospital as a primary source of these data. The fact sheet on the discharge summary of the medical record will include the necessary data. Some hospitals have an abstracting service, which will provide a swift way to obtain such information. All the data you collect, regardless of whether it is for service area, the medical staff, demographics, or so forth, must be up-to-date, accurate, usefully presented and properly interpreted, understandable, and comprehensive.

Some of the facts that a hospital needs to know about the patients they serve include groupings such as the following: where the patients live (sometimes this is done by zip codes, depending upon the size of the community); information about hospital services in obstetrics, pediatrics, intensive care, and so on; source of payment, including Blue Cross, Medicare, and other breakdowns; and admission source, such as elective, urgent, emergency department. Some hospitals divide their service area into primary areas, secondary areas, and tertiary. This is not always very fruitful because such knowledge often has no use or purpose.

In any business you have to know your competition. The relevance index will enable you to be able to compare how you are doing with other hospitals in a given geographic area.

Utilization Trends. Utilization issues cover two broad areas. The first relates to community utilization such as consumption of health care. For example, does your community use 1,400 days per thousand population? Some HMO areas use 600. It is important to compare your community's consumption of health care with national and statewide norms in order to see where you stand relative to other communities. If consumption is high, there will be pressures from state health departments, Blue Cross, and other sources for your hospital to do what it can to reduce consumption. Even the number of beds allowed may be cut back to force a reduction in consumption. You are also interested in your hospital's use rate of obstetrics, surgery, pediatrics, and so forth. Admissions per thousand of population will also be important data for you to obtain.

When you are examining the utilization trends for your hospital for the past five to ten years, one good approach to consider would be to determine the number of beds that your hospital had available in total as well as broken down by service such as pediatrics, obstetrics, neonatology, medical-surgical; then list the percentage of occupancy for each service for each year, as well as number of discharges, the average length of stay, total inpatient days, and so on. In this way you will be able to determine trends in utilization of the facilities of your hospital.

Since the purpose of this entire section is to determine an environmental analysis and since the utilization of our present services is important to assess our environment, this then becomes one of the most important areas of long-range plans. By assimilating these data we can quickly determine what is happening to occupancy levels in such departments as general medicine as well as the subareas, general surgery, and the subspecialties, obstetrics, pediatrics, child psychiatry, and others.

Medical Staff Analysis. In order to prepare a comprehensive environmental analysis, you need to continue your effort to compile important data. One of the key areas that will need to be examined is your medical staff. A great deal of data on the medical staff must be obtained in order to prepare a statement of your hospital's environmental analysis. Planning for the medical staff needs of your hospital is a very essential component of the master plan.

If a particular hospital, for example, is located in the inner city and many of its physicians have moved to the suburbs, and if the occupancy level has been steadily falling downward, it becomes important to ascertain the relationship between the number of physicians on staff and the occupancy rate. A continuing trend like this is likely to result in bankruptcy.

Similarly, a hospital with an average physician age of 59 may have had a stable occupancy rate for several years, but unless new physicians are being brought in, it also may be headed for trouble. In any event, unless you have at least the data about who your physicians are and where they are, you will not be able to prepare a master plan that will be helpful to the future of the hospital.

We have already discussed the importance of involving the medical staff in the planning process. Now you need to examine why the analysis of the medical staff is so important to the future of your hospital. A major element in strategic planning is the role of physicians in marketing their hospital. Marketing should not be left only to the administrators. Trustees, physicians, and others are a key part of a total marketing effort.

Following are some examples of the types of data a hospital needs regarding its physicians: a breakdown by name, age, specialty area, board certification information, type of physician appointment, when they became members of the staff, number of admissions that each physician brought to the hospital during each of the last five years, the percentage of the total admissions of the physician at the hospital for each of the last five years (for example, physicians who are on the staff of three or four hospitals have more flexibility in where they take their patients than if they are on the staff of only your hospital; important data can be derived by examining trends to see if your doctors are *increasingly* bringing patients to your hospital or *increasingly* taking them to other hospitals).

It is one thing to gather all these data, and quite another to analyze them. It is very important for the planning staff to develop the data and to present to the planning committee a comprehensive analysis and interpretation of what the data represents. For example, if a particular obstetrician accounts for 30 percent of all of the obstetric admissions in your hospital and he is 64 years of age, you need a plan for staff recruitment right away.

It is also important to know staff attitudes regarding your hospital. One of the objectives here is to set up a relationship between the services that are being planned for your hospital and the kinds of physician specialists that you presently have and the ones you will need in order to achieve those objectives. All of these issues have to be coordinated.

Obtaining all of these data is no easy task. Your present medical staff files probably will not contain all of this information. Since the obtaining of this information is part of the planning process and since by now you have medical staff representatives on the planning committee, it ought not to be a very difficult task to obtain the support of the executive committee of the medical staff for a comprehensive questionnaire to be distributed among medical staff members to supplement the present data that you have on them. In large hospitals in large cities this might be quite a task indeed, since many staff members may be recalcitrant to fill out a questionnaire and send it in. Much follow-up will be necessary.

In some cities there is information available, through hospitals that have gotten together to share their patient origin information, from which the hospital can obtain the percentages of hospital admissions among various hospitals for their medical staff members. If this is the case where your hospital is located, then you are well on the way to obtaining some of the most dynamic information that is necessary for the planning process.

Individual physicians either may not wish to reveal such data as where they practice, in terms of which hospital, and what percentage of their patients go to which hospital, or they may feel that they are not able to estimate it correctly. In smaller hospitals, especially in rural areas, this data gathering process takes on a different framework because in those instances the importance lies in physician recruitment.

Demographics. Demographics refers to the statistical study of area populations with special reference to the extent of population, location and density, distribution, ethnic origin, employment, income, and education.

The purpose of the demographic analysis is to help you obtain a good understanding of the potential health care needs of the area that you serve. If the income of your population served is going down, then you may have future financial problems in reimbursement. This could affect the future financial viability of your hospital.

Information from the 1970 and 1980 comparative census will be a rich source of dramatic data for this analysis. Most of this information can be obtained from the local council of government, the State Health Planning and Development Agency, urban and regional planning agencies, HSAs, State Office of Management and Budget, and the Bureau of the Census.

After the planning office of your hospital has gathered the information, it should prepare an interpretation report for review by the planning committee. The objective here is to prepare a comprehensive statement of the environmental analysis of your hospital with specific regard to demographics as well as to the other areas covered in this chapter. The actual data are not always important unless you are able to assess trends in what the data show. The analysis of such data will result in your being able to identify special target populations for service.

One of the obvious results of this is that if there is significant population growth, then an increase in the number of beds for your hospital may have to be considered. The fruits of strategic planning become especially significant when data such as these are gathered, interpreted, and presented. Many new programs, such as gerontology, may need to be included in the formulation of objectives as a result of these data.

Health Services Inventory. One of the primary purposes of a health services inventory is to determine what community resources are presently available. By determining this you are able to identify gaps or excesses. For example, what are the needs in the community for mental health services, ambulatory health care delivery, pediatrics, obstetrics, emergency room activity, a burn unit, neonatal intensive care unit, hemodialysis. You will need to estimate a demand for all of these services based upon a health services inventory. You will then be in a position to establish priorities.

Some of this information can be obtained by examining the utilization of present inpatient services. A particular population's health status is strongly affected by life style of the inhabitants. It is very difficult to measure accurately the general health status of the population that you are serving at the hospital.

Some of the basic data that will be covered will include infant mortality, in which trends will be determined from an examination of the data. You should examine the leading causes of death for your service area population. Obtaining such information will help enable you to establish priorities for the kinds of services that you should assimilate to render care to your community. The primary source of such data can be obtained annually from local and state health departments. Your HSA or health department will have some of this information too.

Fertility rates can be determined, as well as illegitimate live births broken down by zip code, service area, county, region, and state. Information should be obtained on selected communicable disease incidences such as tuberculosis and venereal disease. Local hospital councils may also have much of this information. After it is obtained, it should be analyzed and interpreted by the planning staff and presented to the planning committee.

Financial Analysis. The financial resources of your hospital should be examined in a comprehensive manner. This is largely an internal data-gathering step in which the chief financial officer of the hospital will play a major role. Key financial data should be determined for each of the last five years, and trends noted. This would include determination of trends in the following: net operating revenue, excess of revenue over expenses, balance sheet areas, sources of revenue, bad debt accumulation, type of payer mix, operating expenses broken down by wages, benefits, and other major divisions of the hospital. Long- and short-term debts should be analyzed.

Examination should take place of the sources and uses of funds that would be available for program and project development. Some of the areas relative to the historical cost per unit of service such as acute care cost, ancillary cost, and inpatient cost will relate to the data prepared earlier that was available from the medical records department.

Issues and Problems

The preparation of the comprehensive statement of the environmental assessment of your hospital will constitute a major source for the preparation of the statement of issues and problems for your hospital. Another source for information for the statement of issues and problems is a comprehensive interviewing of various key persons in the hospital and the community. Sometimes such interviewing is done by consultants, or it can be done by hospitals' chief planning officers as well as by certain members assisting them from the hospitals' planning staffs.

A specific plan should be outlined detailing where to obtain all of the information for the statement of issues and problems. For example, in regard to interviews, a specific target list should be made, such as all members of the executive committee of the medical staff and a representative sampling of private practitioners and other physicians; all board members; all members of administration; major department heads; and key community representatives such as the head of the local HSA, the head of the local hospital council, state and local health department directors, among others. In addition to having a specific plan for which interviews to conduct, you should also have a list of what questions to ask.

All issues and problems should be conceptualized. The reason is that sometimes a solution is being brought forth when actually you are seeking issues. For example, if your hospital has a high occupancy, the medical staff member may view this as a shortage of beds and will be discussing the lack of beds as the major problem of the hospital; a CEO may view the same information (high occupancy) as an efficient utilization of resources.

Another word of caution is in order concerning the listing of weaknesses. It will be tempting to immediately list all the actions that you feel would assist in alleviating the weaknesses. However, this is not the time to do it. Programs are brought forth later in response to objectives, and this step should not be bypassed. For example, if your emergency department activity is declining and affecting occupancy, you may receive physician pressures to purchase a CT scanner, or pressures may occur that would suggest a construction of an office building for physicians or establishment of executive physical programs. These may be good directions to take, but they must flow from the planning process and not be evaluated prematurely. While alternative strategies and solutions are being developed, a whole range of programs and actions can be developed at that time.

The way that an issue or problem is described will determine and influence the type of solutions and programs that will be investigated. In other words, the key to all of this is that you are seeking issues and problems and not solutions and programs during the interviewing phase of determining a comprehensive statement of issues and problems. One of the reasons that this is so important is that you do not want to limit the range of alternatives that should be explored to remedy any given situation that exists.

All issues and problems brought forth should be stated in a manner that would encourage open dialogue among all members of the planning committee. You will need innovative thinking that will examine entire ranges of possible solutions.

One weakness requiring innovative thinking that exists in many urban hospitals is location in an over-bedded area. Problems can arise from the potential pressures from the community for debedding. In addition, competition tends to increase when hospitals are vying with one another for the filling of their beds. Often closely tied to this is a declining population, which must be addressed by the hospital. Some of the actions that can be taken here would be to establish a satellite ambulatory care center, satellite ambulatory surgery centers, and/or satellite emergency health care centers. These can serve as stakeouts for future expansion or relocation of inpatient beds as well as being feeders to the home hospital.

The location of an urban hospital in an area of decreasing population will tend to result in increasing dependence upon the immediate community for inpatient admissions. A whole set of strategies must then be set in motion to prevent this problem from becoming very serious to future occupancy. The major issue here is that long-term steps need to be established in order to penetrate and create new markets and to improve the hospital's ability to attract new patients.

Hospitals continue to face threats of declines in occupancy for a large number of reasons, not the least of which is the continuing major trend in ambulatory surgery, which tends to reduce occupancy levels; preadmission testing and pressures to reduce average length of stay can also reduce inpatient occupancy levels.

Another example of a weakness is that a hospital may have an insufficient number of family practitioners, pediatricians, and internists to sustain its referral staff; in other words, a hospital may have a large number of subspecialists both in surgery as well as in internal medicine, and then they *must* have a high number of referral physicians to maintain a good balance. In addition, one of the major weaknesses of many urban hospitals is that they may not have the financial resources to take on additional responsibility for providing care for indigent patients. All of these challenges are related to the mission of the hospital and therefore continue to reinforce the importance of strategic planning.

Trend Analysis

All the above information deals primarily with short-term indicators of needed change. But in order to exploit opportunities, you must also appreciate what is happening outside your organization, not only in the immediate environment of customers and competitors but also in the macroenvironment.

Changes in the macroenvironment are crucial to the relevancy of your health care delivery system. If you could send a scout out into the future, receive reports, and ensure your survival by being prepared, it would be tremendously helpful. Of course it is impossible to send someone into the future itself because the future by definition does not exist. However, you can and should explore ideas about the future—conceptions of what might happen. You do this as part of strategic planning by reviewing the work of "futurists," economists and other experts in a variety of fields who describe what they foresee evolving in our macroenvironment by, say, the year 2000.

Here, for example, are some ideas from a collection of such futurists that might give you pause to consider whether you are far-reaching enough in what you include in your strategic planning.

Looking ahead to the year 2000, many experts see an explosion in medical knowledge and technology and further demand for better distribution of quality care and containment of its costs. They are quite certain of dramatic changes, advances—such as genetic counseling and antiviral agents—that will vanquish some of today's worst health scourges and lessen the fearful consequences of others.

We Americans get more and better medical care than in previous generations, and care should continue to improve. But the results from scientific advances are diminishing. Many health authorities believe that more doctors and more hospitals will have no more effect on good health overall than the way people live. The next major advance in the health of the American people will result only from what the individual is willing to do for himself or herself.

The most significant change in the future of medicine may very well be a shift in health care delivery system from our present "physician-centered" system to a "medic–computer" system, in which computers will render most of the technical, diagnostic, and treatment decisions while medics provide supportive tasks, both technical and emotional. This shift will provide patients with both technically and humanistically superior medical care. Medical technology and health care will be increasingly affected by computerized medicine, which will not only speed the assimilation of knowledge but also improve the cost and efficiency of health care. Computers already perform a variety of tasks in hospitals but in the future they will likely provide greater services in:

- automated medical records to ensure coordination among health care personnel
- patient examination to analyze everything from vision to lungs to blood chemistry and transmit such information from home to office to hospital
- diagnosis to match symptoms and outcomes from centralized data bases

We will probably witness changing patterns of illness rather than complete elimination of disease. As the average life span increases, we encounter disorders associated with older age—cancer, stroke, heart disease, and so forth. Between 1980 and 2000 we will learn how to better treat and control these specific diseases. Future disorders expected to increase in frequency are emphysema, arthritic disorders, aging, and antisocial behavior (as we become more isolated from one another psychologically).

Over the next 20 years, biomedical engineering will improve and expand organ transplants, genetic modification, mind and behavior modification, and reproductive techniques. Some of the major technological advances to be researched and their implications include:

- amniocentesis—a prenatal procedure to examine for genetic disorders, which will diminish incidences of genetically defective births, cause a reevaluation of health care and insurance procedure, and present the dilemma of individual freedom of decision for social reasons (for example, abort or risk having a defective child)
- cloning—asexual propagation, which will revolutionize notions of mortality, individuality, reproduction, sex, marriage, and hundreds of other concepts and institutions; knowledgeable scientists predict human cloning will be a reality by 1995
- biofeedback—an awareness of bodily functions that will lead to a new understanding of mind and body relationship, less dependence on drugs, and a reassessment of basic beliefs about medicine
- psychosurgery—brain modification, the ability to experience sensations at will, which will alter personality and open countless ethical questions
- cryogenics—life extension by animation, by drugs, or by enclosure in vacuum containers, which will prolong both animal and plant life and also open countless ethical questions.
- cyborgs—replacement of human organs with durable equipment, which will prompt a reordering of our health sciences, the whole life cycle, and almost every institution
- man–computer combinations—tiny computers implanted in the human brain to boost memory and intelligence, perhaps to remedy hereditary or chronic brain deficiencies

Life expectancy in 1900 was 47.3 years, and in 1980 it was 74 years. By the year 2025, it will be 85 years. Advances in diagnosis and treatment or prevention of cardiovascular diseases, cerebrovascular diseases, and cancer; organ transplant and development of nonbiologic prostheses; and improvements in life style and environment will account for much of this increase. All of these considerations ought to raise numerous questions regarding alternatives for your organization's strategic planning consistent with your mission.

So far we should have some kind of agreement as to strengths and weaknesses so there will be a common understanding of our starting point for setting objectives. Remember, we are at a certain point in time, which is related to other points in the recent past: we are not standing still waiting for a chance to set an objective for the future. We are on our way somewhere whether we have defined that point yet or not. We are always caught up in some sort of momentum because our present position reflects recent trends. It will be helpful, therefore, to be aware of the trends, of the forces we now face, of the direction we have been going, either forward or backward (winning or losing) in at least certain key areas.

The areas chosen are often considered the seven key functional concerns of any CEO, so you are now role-playing the position of CEO and should be concerned about these key areas. In a typical hospital, they might be the areas of operations, quality of care, finance, productivity, public relations, growth in services, and personnel.

When asking for the views of each participant in the group, you will not only be seeking a consensus as to where you are, but you will also help resolve differences. You want to know whether you are going forward or backward (winning or losing) by asking each person, "as measured by what?"

You are doing two things here. First, you are showing it is possible for one person to say "winning" and another to say "losing" about the same item, though both can be correct and compatible because each is using something different as the yardstick for making the judgment. Second, you are deliberately seeking to know what yardsticks different persons use to make judgments, even if they arrive at the same conclusion relative to winning or losing.

Taking the seven key areas in turn, let's look at some of the considerations that frequently arise with each of them, see an example, and then complete this part of the exercise for your unit.

1. Are you winning or losing in number or percent of those served? This is the *volume of business* area. While you are concerned with occupancy or volume of procedures, you ought also to be concerned with the marketability of your service in terms of whether you are reaching those you should. In other words, this (and other questions) asks you to make judgments not only in terms of what you are doing but also in terms of what you should be doing.

   When you get to a particular division or department, you might find you should be concerned about your service not only to patients but also to other departments of the hospital. Are you winning or losing there, perhaps as measured by the complaints from those departments?

Question: Make your judgments regarding the current trend in the area of those served, with emphasis on "as measured by what."

Answer:

2. Are you winning or losing in the superiority of your patient care or service? This is the *quality control* function. Obviously there is some overlap with the previous question, because now you are trying to make a judgment about what you offer to those you serve. The discussion will naturally get involved not only with what you offer them, but also what they think of your services.

   This is frequently the most embarrassing section of needs analysis. There is a tendency for hospitals to be proud of their service, even though they are not quite so able to describe what it is that makes their patient care or service superior. What aspect of your service do you feel stands out? What can you offer that others cannot? How have you responded to the felt needs of those you serve? What testing devices do you use to check on quality of services you offer year after year? Can you point to innovative programs? Can you cite special honors or recognitions? Or, are you aware of places where quality has fallen down? What was learned during the last regular audit or JCAH visitation?

Question: List your judgments regarding current trends in the superiority of services. As always, the crucial information sought is what measures winning or losing.

Answer:

3. Are you winning or losing in your financial condition? This is the *finance* function and has already been discussed in this chapter.

   Some component units will find they are revenue producers, and others will find they are strictly cost centers. How each sees itself fiscally accountable will come out in the course of the discussion at this time. (Very often the willingness of the top manager to share financial information is tested here. Participation in the decision-making process requires sufficient information to give an informed opinion about the decision, and finances usually are an important part of that background.)

Question: Evaluate your financial condition. Share insights and methods of measuring progress in this key area.

Answer:

4. Are you winning or losing in the area of productivity of staff? This is the *efficiency* function. Every effort should be made to consider productivity not only in the classic accounting manner of "number of units of output divided by number of man-hours worked" but also in the full sense of total output divided by *all* the factors of production, all inputs (i.e., labor, land, and capital).

   Our recent national and international inflationary spiral has brought about a wide awareness of the need for all segments of the economy (not only business) to face up to the challenge of increasing productivity. Whether we produce and sell widgets or provide patient care, we must find ways of spreading the world's resources further. (You will recall here the discussion in Chapter 1 about MBO seeking to keep the correct relationship between inputs and outputs.) Exhibit 5-2 shows how productivity was judged in our sample hospital.

Question: Are you winning or losing in your productivity? Include the various ways of measuring the normal work output.

Answer:

5. Are you winning or losing in the area of public opinion? This is the *public relations* function. It is the area in which you tend to find great

Exhibit 5-2 Sample Ways to Measure Productivity

Department	*Unit*
Nursing	
Nursing Administration and Unit Services	Hrs/total patient days
Pediatric-Teens	Hrs/patient day
Obstetrics	Hrs/patient day
Intensive Care Unit	Hrs/patient day
Medical–Surgical	Hrs/patient day
Coronary Care Unit	Hrs/patient day
TOTAL	Hrs/patient day
Nursery	Hrs/patient day
Operating Room	Man-hrs/procedure
PAR	Man-hrs/surg anes
Emergency Room	Man-hrs/procedure
Delivery Room	Man-hrs/delivery
Service Managers	Man-hrs/patient day
Laboratory	Procedures/man-hrs
EKG	Tests/100 man-hrs
EEG	Tests/100 man-hrs
Radiology	Man-hrs/procedure
Radioisotope	Tests/100 man-hrs
Pharmacy	Rx/man-hr*
Anesthesia	Anesthetics/100 man-hrs
Physical Therapy	Treatments/man-hrs
Medical Records	Man-hrs/discharge
Dietary	Meals/man-hrs
Business Office	Man-hrs/discharge
Admitting Office	Man-hrs/admission
Housekeeping	Man-hrs/1000 sq ft/mo

* Includes intravenous therapy at equivalent of 7 to 1

differences because there are so many "publics" to be considered. Where do you stand with your employees, patients, or suppliers? The broad public (meaning the civil community)—how do you stand with your local citizens, especially the taxpaying ones? What about the press and other mass media? They constitute a public also. Are you winning or losing with your competitors, your associations, and the governmental or regulatory agencies?

Question: Complete such a list of judgments and ways of measuring by seeking contributions from all. What do they think of your public opinion? If you think of a way of measuring but do not know what the answer would be, this should not be lost, but put aside for possible use in setting objectives.

Answer:

6. Are you winning or losing in vitality (*growth of services*)? How are you doing on creativity? Are you responding to new needs? Are you progressive or conservative? Do you foster innovation? Do you listen? Do you engage in research? What do your vital signs say: are you healthy or falling apart?

Question: What do you think about vitality? How do you measure this important aspect of any unit? Are you well or sick? Are you alive? Does anyone care? How do you know?

Answer:

7. Are you winning or losing in personal development and other personnel issues? This is really the *career planning* function. Do you have career plans? Are there back-up people (actual or in preparation) for key positions? Do you deliberately plan movements of people by preparing them for new jobs? Are you recruiting the way you should be? Are you looking to the future to cover expansion plans with adequate human resources? Do you provide good inservice? Are you a teaching institution?

Question: What direction are you going in personnel administration: up or down? As measured by what? Remember it is as important to list ways of measurement as anything else.

Answer:

Although there is no prescribed format, we will now describe an example of what a statement of issues and problems could look like.

Our Image

1. The majority of interviews conducted have indicated that our hospital is looked upon as an "inner city" hospital with a good track

record in serving the poor. There is disagreement about the emphasis we should give to tertiary care versus being a community general hospital with an emphasis on service to the immediate neighborhoods.
2. The hospital needs more "exciting" services.
3. Patients are often reluctant to come to our hospital because of fear of safety.

Service Area

1. Many of our former patients have left for the suburbs, and this trend appears to be continuing.
2. Most patients in our hospital who live in the community nearby use the emergency room for their source of care, and this means that many of our patients do not get continuity in their medical care.
3. Since our service area population served is shifting in various communities near the hospital, what can we do to stabilize or to shape it?

Medical Staff

1. Most of our medical staff have left the immediate surroundings of the hospital to move into suburbia.
2. Some attending staff physicians do not feel committed to the service of patients in our immediate neighborhoods and feel that the hospital is giving too much attention to the areas adjacent to the hospital.
3. There is a high average age in primary care departments, including general practice and obstetrics.
4. There are decreasing admission trends in the surgical subspecialty areas.
5. Some clinical areas are much stronger than others.
6. In the past five years, over 90 percent of our 100 house staff have been foreign medical graduates, and now the trend is increasing to a higher number.
7. Some residency programs are so weak that they may not be approved in the next evaluation.

Demographic Factors

1. Population in our primary service area is decreasing, and the population in our secondary area is increasing.
2. Our geriatric population is increasing faster than the general population.

Health Status

1. Problems in the 1980s will not relate to general health but will be caused more by behavioral and environmental factors.

2. Underserved persons will continue to have problems in access to continuity of care.
3. The incidence of chronic disease is moving upward; some of the high rates of disease are in heart disease, alcohol and drug abuse, and cancer.
4. There will be a lack of outreach programs to meet the needs of the underserved.

Government—Third Party Payers

1. The role of the federal government is mixed at the present time; during the 1970s it was predicted that the government's role would increasingly dominate the delivery and financing of health care services; in the 1980s the role of deregulation may occur, national health services are not likely, at least until 1988, and the government's impact on reimbursement, rather than regulation of health care, may be the major role that will be taken by the federal government.
2. Restrictive reimbursement policies will make it increasingly difficult for hospitals to continue their increase of services to the health care community; special strategies will be necessary to live within budgets.

Miscellaneous

1. There will be more competition among hospitals and throughout health care, and this will place many challenges on our hospitals.
2. Our inadequate parking facilities, which are short by over 400 cars, will place many problems on us unless solutions are brought forth.
3. Our hospital needs to have more concern over the future of the city and the problem that the city faces.
4. Even with high unemployment we will face challenges in recruitment of certain skilled professionals, particularly registered nurses.
5. There will be challenges to religious and ethical positions on such issues as the right to die with dignity and the right to refuse treatment.

Priorities. After your planning committee has assembled a draft of the issues and problems facing your hospital, the next step is to prioritize all the issues and problems so that you will have an ordering of your future direction. What you have done so far is to isolate the issues that are a legitimate part of your long-range planning process; now these parts have to be prioritized. One of the best ways to do this is to have the planning committee appoint a subcommittee to recommend a prioritization of the issues, and the subcommittee will meet two or three times to complete this task and then submit its recommendations to the overall planning committee. They should be submitted well ahead of time so that the members can examine them before going over the recommended prioritization at one or two subsequent planning committee meetings.

Involvement here is very important. Input should be sought from all members of the board as well as the executive committee of the medical staff and members of administration. Some of that coordinative effort can be done by the ad-hoc committee that will be recommending the prioritization of the issues. The greater the involvement, the greater will be the tendency for the members of the hospital's family to own the document when it is finally completed!

Following are some of the criteria that the planning committee can use in ascertaining priorities: Is there anything the hospital can really do about a particular issue or will it have to enlist the assistance of others in order to have a potential impact? How severe is each problem? Can the severity of the problem be measured in terms of quality of life? How major is each problem in regard to how many persons are affected or how many hospital programs or services are affected? What would be the expected consequences of each problem or issue if nothing were done regarding it? For example, would the problem or issue improve by itself or would it become significantly worse?

A section on problems and issues must be carefully documented and must be updated at least annually. If several years go by without updating this section, the long-range plan will become out-of-date. The momentum of your hospital must be maintained. You cannot stop and rest. Movement that is not forward will be backward.

SUMMARY

The end of your planning responsibilities as board member, CEO, or physician does not come when you have put your strategic plan in writing. Listen to the definition of the strategic plan given by the Stanford Research Institute:

> The strategic plan is the long-term means which top management uses to guide an organization toward a desired future position. This plan determines the nature and scope of all other plans and reaches beyond them in time.

This suggests that a state of strategic thinking is needed; the plan should never be frozen or the process considered over. Hence, your hospital should be characterized continuously by:

- a sensitivity to the environment in which it functions, specifically in terms of the threats and opportunities that environment offers
- a clear definition of the mission of your hospital, which states the purpose of the organization in the light of changing societal needs
- a concrete statement of the objectives it wishes to attain and that are possible for it to attain
- a detailed itemization of the action steps necessary to respond to the major issues involved in realizing objectives, which will include such things as resource development and deployment and assignment of accountabilities

Some of this will be foreign to the way you have conducted business in the past. Some of it will bring to your attention the possibility of changes that may make future medical practice, future health care delivery, future health administration so different that you wouldn't recognize them, and therefore you may wish to close such pictures out of your mind.

But such is the nature of changing society and such must be the nature of your practices if you wish to keep up with society, keeping in mind something written by the philosopher poet Ralph Waldo Emerson:

> A mind, stretched by a new idea, never returns to its original shape.

NOTES

1. David E. Ross, "Planning for Survival in Small and Rural Hospitals," *Hospitals*, June 16, 1980, p. 69.
2. Richard Chaite, "Mission Madness Strikes Our Colleges," *The Chronicle of Higher Education*, July 16, 1979.
3. Ross, "Small and Rural Hospitals," p. 65.
4. See American Hospital Association, "Environmental Assessment of the Hospital Industry, 1979," Chicago, 1979.
5. See Exhibit 5-2.

Appendix 5-A

Sample Mission Statements of Hospital Departments

MISSION STATEMENT FOR AN AMBULATORY CARE CENTER

As one of the major operational units of this not–for-profit community general hospital, the mission of the ambulatory care unit is to provide high-quality care and services on an outpatient basis to residents and visitors of __(city)__ who comprise the primary target population of __________________ Hospital. Major programs currently include a diagnostic clinic, 20 specialty clinics and diagnostic and therapeutic services, and the short-stay surgery program.

We are committed to continuous assessment of the changing demand for ambulatory services by the people of our community and to the development of appropriate services and programs that will both respond to recognized needs and stimulate awareness of unrecognized needs for preventive and curative health care.

We are dedicated to maintaining our position of leadership in ambulatory care by vigorously promoting innovative programs for the sick and the well, while fostering cost-containment principles and practices such as cooperation with other ambulatory care providers within our service area, as well as with local health care planners, to develop and implement an areawide ambulatory referral system based on level of care needed.

MISSION STATEMENT FOR GENERAL SUPPORT SERVICES

The role of the General Support division is to provide support services that facilitate accomplishment of the hospital mission. Our basic purpose is to supply and protect the hospital's assets and to provide certain centralized, specialized services. In order to achieve excellence in patient care, education and research, flexibility, creativity, willingness, dependability, stability, and consistency are all necessary attributes. We are committed to maximizing the efficiency of the hospital staff, especially the medical and patient care staff.

We are committed to a leadership position in the field of material service. To do this we must consider the total needs of parents, family, and staff when requests are made. By communicating our involvement in the physical, emotional, spiritual, and psychological needs of our customers, we provide a comforting function to the organization. This comfort engenders and fosters the trust of our customers. We are therefore committed to an extensive pediatric clinical and biomedical knowledge base for paramedical problem solving.

We are committed to a total systems approach to support services. We maintain a constant state of readiness including the ability to anticipate needs. We must respond to special and emergency situations without notice. We strive never to say "No."

We are committed to cost-effectiveness both in our operation and in the operation of other departments. We feel that we have a special role in supporting the risk management program in our supply and equipment acquisition program.

We are a developing division and therefore put great emphasis on both people and system development, especially as it affects the paramedical materiel operations.

MISSION STATEMENT FOR PURCHASING DEPARTMENT

The mission of the Purchasing Department is to provide the highest quality products and services for the hospital and its component units at the most competitive price. We are committed to minimizing costs, which ultimately must be paid by patients or other responsible parties, but not at the risk of poor quality, unreliable service, or inability to provide our health care practitioners with reasonable equipment and supplies.

MISSION STATEMENT FOR NURSING SERVICE

To maximize quality patient care and foster professional development of our staff is the purpose of the Nursing Service Division. This will include effective programs for patient care procedures, for nursing care plans, for cooperation with other health care practitioners, for outgoing professional training, and for efficient utilization of hospital resources.

MISSION STATEMENT FOR VOLUNTEER SERVICES DEPARTMENT

The Volunteer Services Department plans and coordinates a program of volunteer services directly supporting the purpose and objectives of this hospital. It is dedicated to serving the hospital by recruiting, selecting, and developing the many types of volunteer resources and activities necessary to fulfill the hospital's mission.

Many types of people in the area are willing to work for free at this hospital. They include students, housewives, senior citizens, and professionals who would like to donate their time and talents. Their motives are many: some wish to help sick children, others need work experience or school credit, some have a lot of free time and want something interesting to do with it.

Our philosophy is that volunteers have special talents and skills that should be recognized in assigning them a job in a specific hospital department, thus enabling them to make a greater contribution, since continuity and training integrates them into the hospital staff.

The Volunteer Services Department was organized to assist department managers in taking advantage of this resource. It serves as a "personnel office" for volunteers and coordinates their activities in the hospital. However, volunteers are supervised not by the volunteer coordinator, but by the volunteer chairperson of each activity. This chairperson reports to the department manager, who is responsible for the success of volunteer activities within the department.

MISSION STATEMENT FOR UTILIZATION REVIEW

The Utilization Review Section is charged with the continuous review in our hospital of our pattern of services, particularly the necessity of certain services of a sample of patients based on age-sex-diagnostic criteria, as a means of making recommendations.

In carrying out its duties, this section shall evaluate the appropriateness of admissions on an inpatient basis, the length of stay of the patient, discharge and transfer practices, services to be rendered, and all other related factors that may contribute to effective utilization of our hospital facilities.

The utilization review section is committed to maintaining JCAH and PSRO standards and ensuring that all patients receive necessary, appropriate, and effective medical, nursing, and other forms of direct patient care.

MISSION STATEMENT FOR MEDICAL RECORDS DEPARTMENT

The Medical Records Department has the ongoing responsibility of developing, maintaining, and coordinating all information within the hospital relating to patient care and services. We are the clearinghouse and custodian of all official documentation regarding patients.

This department creates, updates, contributes to, audits, completes, and safeguards the patient's chart. It is our primary duty to oversee the adequacy, correctness, and timeliness of patient records and ensure that quality standards as determined by regulatory agencies, administration, and professional groups are maintained.

In so doing, we assist quality of care in a fourfold way: through reporting, monitoring, auditing, and predicting. These activities assist both management and professional staff in establishing and maintaining a premier level of excellence of patient care, education, and research activities.

MISSION STATEMENT FOR PASTORAL CARE DEPARTMENT

The mission of the Department of Pastoral Care is to provide, through the "religious presence" of the staff, an environment in which patients, significant others, and staff can experience and be strengthened by the healing power of Christ. This mission is accomplished through both the sacramental and pastoral care ministry.

Future programs that will give the pastoral care staff greater patient contact include: initial visit program; involvement in preop group to meet patients and thereby evaluate their needs and respond with appropriate pastoral ministry; a program to encourage the reception of the anointing of the sick; religious information and education program using closed circuit television; and inservice education for doctors and nurses in the role of pastoral care in crisis intervention and grief.

Programs to increase the community's awareness of the mission of the hospital will involve: seminars for clergy and laity relating to religious-medical topics; religious education in conjunction with local clergy for the laity of the area; and continued awareness of the needs of the community and an appropriate response to those needs.

MISSION STATEMENT FOR NUCLEAR MEDICINE DEPARTMENT

The mission of the Department of Nuclear Medicine and Computed Tomography is to provide the patient and the physician with the most modern and beneficial diagnostic and therapeutic procedures that are available today. Modern instrumentation and progressive techniques will be utilized while attempting to minimize the increasing costs relative to these fields.

Within the next five years the Department of Nuclear Medicine and Computed Tomography will undergo many changes. Within the next year we hope to have achieved a departmental relocation to a more workable area, and by the end of the budget year to have reacquired new nuclear medicine equipment to replace the present leased equipment.

We hope to upgrade the EMI scanner to fast scan capabilities if indicated or necessary. We also will constantly be on the lookout for any new progressive instrumentation that will provide better health care to the patient at the hospital.

MISSION STATEMENT FOR PATIENT CARE DIVISION OF A CHILDREN'S HOSPITAL

The Patient Care Department is dedicated to ensuring qualified competent care in restoring, maintaining, and enhancing the health and recovery of children and the support to their families. In the process of administering diagnostic and treatment services, we create an atmosphere conducive to maximizing the child's growth and development.

Through established standards of care, we provide comprehensive health care to meet each patient's needs. The patient care plan will reflect the physical, spiritual, emotional, social, and developmental needs, and the patient's rights as an individual. To ensure the quality of care, we continually evaluate and update the plan of care and establish monitoring programs such as audits, risk management, and other effective reporting systems. Because our efforts are centered on the total patient's needs, we place special emphasis on the importance of play and a safe environment.

Recognizing that the patient is an integral part of a family unit, we strive to meet the needs of the parents and family to maintain as much as possible their unity during his/her hospitalization. This also provides the staff an ongoing opportunity to communicate, prepare, teach, and assist the family for the care requirements of the child after discharge.

To effectively plan for the child's discharge, we act as a liaison between the hospital, other institutions, and community resources available for preventive and follow-up care.

To ensure an effective system of patient care, we commit ourselves to the development of a professional staff by encouraging attendance at educational and clinical programs on a continuous basis. We promote participation in leadership programs, research opportunities, and sharing of creative/innovative ideas through publication. We encourage suggestions and participation of staff in planning and implementing short- and long-term goals of our institution.

The Patient Care Division (including the patient units, departments of nursing education, patient education and recreation, pharmacy, patient services, and respiratory care) recognizes that it is only through the cooperative team efforts of all hospital and medical center departments that we are able to provide care at a reasonable cost.

MISSION STATEMENT FOR A PHARMACY DEPARTMENT

The mission of the Pharmacy Department at ________________ Hospital is to procure, store, and dispense high quality medications to patients in a safe manner while exercising reasonable cost-containment practices. Further, the Pharmacy Department disseminates information on drugs to the medical staff while teaching the nursing staff and patients about drugs.

The Pharmacy Department already has established unit dose and I.V. additives and is anticipating computerization within the year. Over the next five years the Pharmacy Department will focus its energies into the area of inservice education to nurses, patient education on drug regimen compliance, and clinical pharmacy. The pharmacists will be spending more time in the patient care areas attempting to provide information and education to the patient, nurse, and physician, thus further defining their role on the health care team.

MISSION STATEMENT FOR THE PSYCHIATRIC NURSING UNIT

The mission of the Psychiatric Unit is to provide intensive treatment for acute psychiatric illness. The treatment is based on a crisis intervention model using an individualized treatment plan. The goal of treatment is to alleviate the patient's symptoms as rapidly as possible so that the patient can return to the community with minimal disruption of the patient's life.

The Psychiatric Unit is organized in a milieu that respects the patient's independence and provides an environment where treatment is provided by a team approach using social work, nursing, and activity therapy. The Psychiatric Unit is dedicated to providing the highest quality of care and to utilizing all currently acceptable psychiatric treatments that can be helpful to the individual patient.

MISSION STATEMENT FOR THE HUMAN RESOURCES GROUP

The Human Resources Group is dedicated to serving __________ __________ Hospital by assisting in the recruitment, selection, and development of the many types of voluntary and paid human resources necessary for the hospital to fulfill its mission.

In selecting these resources we strive to match the qualifications of the individual with the requirements of the job and at the same time offer opportunity for fulfilling the goals the individual set in joining our organization. Once on the job, we seek to assist the organization and the individual to grow by offering a complete initial orientation program and appropriate internal and external educational and training opportunities. We believe in an organizational climate that demands fair and consistent treatment of all individuals, allows participation in decision making, and views recognition of the performance of its human resources as being essential. By encouraging communication between all levels of human resources within our hospital, by maintaining competitive, equitable, and understandable wages and benefit programs, and by assuming the role of employee advocate, we feel an organizational climate is created in which presence of an outside bargaining representative is unnecessary.

We also recognize the important role we play in the maintenance of a safe healthful environment. In addition we are aware of our responsibility to keep required records and other appropriate data and to provide informational services to the hospital about its human resources. We also are charged with the responsibility of ensuring the organization's compliance with the provisions of various government regulations concerning the organization's human resources. Through the application of appropriate work measurement techniques, we also play a major part in promoting improved productivity in labor utilization and overall cost containment.

Finally we are committed to maintaining a leadership position in human resource areas.

Appendix 5-B

Recommendations for Maintaining a Planning Information System

This section contains a brief series of recommendations designed to facilitate the development, maintenance, and continual refinement of a planning information system at your hospital.

Also included in this section is a table identifying the base data for hospital planning.

RECOMMENDATIONS

- The necessary resources should be made available to the director of planning to maintain and continually refine an information system for the purposes of planning at your hospital.
- The director of planning should work with personnel in the business office, medical records department, and other departments of the hospital to establish the mechanism for routinely collecting information pertinent to planning, which is currently being generated internally. The specific elements of data, the format for recording these data, and the timetable for providing this information to the planning department should be established.
- The director of planning should identify any additional elements of data necessary for planning purposes, which are not currently being collected internally, and should recommend new record-keeping procedures to facilitate the collection of this information.
- The director of planning should attempt to institute a mechanism for information exchange among local providers, involving data and information pertinent to community health area planning.
- The director of planning should establish good working relationships with individuals in the research or statistics divisions of the local and

state health departments, the HSA, the State Health Planning and Development Agency, and local medical schools and universities.

- The director of planning should summarize and display pertinent data through charts, graphs or tables; highlight significant trends and patterns reflected by the data; and develop analyses and conclusions for the benefit of the long-range planning committee.
- The director of planning should update base data and revise projections and analyses as new information becomes available and should ensure that all copies of the data source book are updated and revised as necessary.
- The hospital should initiate special studies in cooperation with other hospitals and health care institutions to identify specific service area health status problems or to determine specific health service needs/demand.

Base Data for Hospital Planning

Type of Data	*Basic Elements*	*Frequency of Collection*	*Primary Source*	*Secondary Source*
I. Repetitive Data				
Inpatient Statistics	Bed complement by clinical service Adult medical Adult surgical Pediatrics Obstetrics Psychiatric Continuing care Critical care units (ICU and CCU)	Quarterly	Business Office	
	Five-year trends (beds)	Annually	Hospital Planning Dept.	
	Patient days by clinical service	Monthly	Medical Record Dept.	Business Office
	Five-year trends (pt. days)	Annually	Hospital Planning Dept.	
	Admissions (discharges) by clinical service	Monthly	Medical Record Dept.	Business Office
	Five-year trends (Adm.)	Annually	Hospital Planning Dept.	
	Occupancy by clinical service	Monthly	Medical Record Dept.	Business Office
	Five-year trends (Occ.)	Annually	Hospital Planning Dept.	
	Average daily census by clinical service	Monthly	Medical Record Dept.	Business Office
	Five-year trends (ADC)	Annually	Hospital Planning Dept.	
	Length of stay by clinical service	Monthly	Medical Record Dept.	Business Office
	Five-year trends (LOS)	Annually	Hospital Planning Dept.	

Type of Data	*Basic Elements*	*Frequency of Collection*	*Primary Source*	*Secondary Source*
	Percentage of total admissions by clinical service	Quarterly	Medical Record Dept.	Business Office
	Percentage of total patient days by clinical service	Quarterly	Medical Record Dept.	Business Office
	Age and sex of patients by clinical service (males–females 0–14, 15–44, 45–64, 65+)	Quarterly	Medical Record Dept.	
	Number of admitting physicians by clinical service	Quarterly	Medical Record Dept.	
	Percent of admission by physician by clinical service	Quarterly	Medical Record Dept.	
	Emergency admissions by clinical service	Quarterly	Medical Record Dept.	
	Referrals to: Home care Nursing home Rehabilitation program Other hospital	Annually	Medical Record Dept.	
	Source of payment by clinical service	Annually	Business Office	
Outpatient Statistics	Emergency room visits Total By source of Referral	Monthly	Medical Record Dept. or Business Office	
	% ER visits admitted	Monthly	Medical Record Dept.	
	% ER visits nonemergent	Monthly	Medical Record Dept.	
	Number of ER patients	Annually	Medical Record Dept. or Business Office	
	Number of ER patients by zipcode	Annually	Medical Record Dept. or Business Office	
	Outpatient clinic visits (Main site and Sumpter)			
	Total	Monthly	Medical Record Dept.	Business Office
	By source referral	Monthly	Medical Record Dept.	
	By clinic	Monthly	Medical Record Dept.	
	By age and sex	Quarterly	Medical Record Dept.	
	By source of payment	Quarterly	Medical Record Dept.	
	Number of patients by outpatient clinic	Annually	Medical Record Dept.	Business Office
	Number of clinic patients by zipcode	Annually	Medical Record Dept. or Business Office	
Supportive/ Ancillary Service Statistics	Laboratory:			
	Inpatient exams	Quarterly	Lab Dept.	
	Exams/inpatient adm.	Annually	Lab Dept.	Business Office
	Clinic exams	Quarterly	Lab Dept.	
	Exams/clinic visit	Annually	Lab Dept.	Business Office
	Outpatient exams	Quarterly	Lab Dept.	

Type of Data	*Basic Elements*	*Frequency of Collection*	*Primary Source*	*Secondary Source*
	Exams/outpatient visit	Annually	Lab Dept.	Business Office
	Total exams	Quarterly	Lab Dept.	
	Exams/man-hour	Quarterly	Lab Dept.	Business Office
	Radiology (Diagnostic):			
	Inpatient studies	Quarterly	Radiology Dept.	
	Studies/admission	Annually	Radiology Dept.	Business Office
	Clinic studies	Quarterly	Radiology Dept.	
	Studies/clinic visit	Annually	Radiology Dept.	Business Office
	Outpatient studies	Quarterly	Radiology Dept.	
	Studies/outpt. visit	Annually	Radiology Dept.	Business Office
	Total studies	Quarterly	Radiology Dept.	
	Studies/man-hour	Quarterly	Radiology Dept.	Business Office
	Surgery:			
	Inpatient operations	Monthly	Surgical Dept.	
	Operations/M/S adm.	Monthly	Surgical Dept.	
	Outpatient operation	Monthly	Surgical Dept.	
	Total operations	Monthly	Surgical Dept.	
	Pharmacy:			
	Line items/man-hour	Quarterly	Pharmacy Dept.	Business Office
	Line items/patient day	Quarterly	Pharmacy Dept.	Business Office
	Physical Therapy:			
	Inpatient treatments	Quarterly	Physical Therapy Dept.	
	Treatments/M/S adm.	Annually	Physical Therapy Dept.	
	Outpatient treatments	Quarterly	Physical Therapy Dept.	
	Treatments/M/S adm.	Annually	Physical Therapy Dept.	Business Office
	Total treatments	Quarterly	Physical Therapy Dept.	
	Social Work:			
	Inpatient interviews by clinical service	Quarterly	Social Work Dept.	
	Interviews/admission by clinical service	Annually	Social Work Dept.	Business Office
	Outpatient interviews	Quarterly	Social Work Dept.	
	ER			
	Clinic			
	Total interviews	Quarterly	Social Work Dept.	
Manpower:	Nursing:			
	FTE by clinic	Quarterly	Nursing	Business Office
	Total service			
	By classification (RN, LPN, Aide)			
	Man-hours/patient day by clinical service	Quarterly	Nursing	Business Office
	Medical Staff:			
	Type of appointment	Annually	Survey	
	Total			
	By Med. Staff Dept.		Survey	
	Five-year trends		Hospital Planning Dept.	
	Age Distribution:	Annually	Survey	
	Total staff			
	By Med. Staff Dept.			
	Five-year trends			
	Specialty Distribution:	Annually	Survey	
	Nonboard			
	Certified			
	Total staff			

Type of Data	*Basic Elements*	*Frequency of Collection*	*Primary Source*	*Secondary Source*
	By Med. Staff Dept. Board certified Total Staff By Med. Staff Dept.			
	Office Location: Number of offices Primary office by zipcode Zipcode map identifying Total med. staff dist.	Annually	Survey	
	Appointments: Number and percent of total staff both joint appts. by major institutions Teaching appointments by Medical Staff Dept.	Annually	Survey	
	Admissions by Physician To Oakwood % Physicians total admissions to any hospital	Annually	Medical Records	
Medical Education	Residency Programs: Available positions Positions filled	Annually	Medical Educ. Dept. or Area Health Educ. Organization	
	Paraprofession Programs: Number of students	Annually	Medical Educ. Dept.	
	Continuing Educ. Programs: Number participants internally Number participants from outside	Annually	Medical Educ. Dept.	
II. Periodic Data				
Service Area Population	Zipcode relevance indices by clinical service	Annually	HSA	Local hospital council
	Percent total Oakwood admissions by clinical service by zipcode	Annually	Hospital Planning Dept.	
	Trends in relevance indices by clinical service by zipcode	Annually/ Biennially	Hospital Planning Dept.	HSA/local hospital council
	Identify service area overlap with other hospitals	Biennially	HSA	Local hospital council
	Define boundaries for primary and secondary service areas and develop zipcode maps for each clinical service	Biennially/ Triennially	Hospital Planning Dept.	Local hospital council

Type of Data	*Basic Elements*	*Frequency of Collection*	*Primary Source*	*Secondary Source*
Demographic Data:	Total Zipcode Population:			
	Individual zipcodes	Annually	Local Council of Governments	
	Aggregate zipcodes	Annually	State Health Planning and Development Agency (SHPDA)	State Office of Development and Budget
	Sex distribution (number & percent) by zipcode, service area, region & state	Triennially	A-95 Urban/Regional Planning Agencies	Dept. of Labor/ Commerce
	Zipcode age distribution (number & percent 0–14, 15–44, 45–64, and 65+) by zipcode, service area, region and state	Triennially		
	Oakwood Service Area Zipcode Population:			
	Individual zipcode contributions to service area populations clinical service (RI × total zipcode pop)	Annually	Hospital Planning Dept.	
	Total service area populations by clinical service (aggregate of zipcode R.I. × zipcode population)	Annually	Hospital Planning Dept.	
	% change in total zipcode population between last census year and base year	Triennially	State Health Planning and Development Agency (SHPDA) and/or State Office of Management and Budget	Local council of governments Dept. of Labor/ Commerce Urban/regional planning agencies (A-95)
	Projected change in zipcode populations between base year and planning years	Triennially	Same as above	Same as above
	Ethnic and racial composition by zipcode, service area, region and state	Decennially (periodic revisions if available)	Bureau of the Census	
	Socioeconomic characteristics by zipcode, service area, region and state:	Decennially (periodic revisions if available)	Bureau of the Census	
	Median income			
	% families below poverty level		Bureau of the Census	
	% families with incomes > $15,000		Bureau of the Census	
	% population 25 years or older with 4 years high school or more		Bureau of the Census	
Health Status Indicators:	Natality Data:			
	Total number of live births by zipcode,	Annually	Local or state health departments	HSA

Type of Data	*Basic Elements*	*Frequency of Collection*	*Primary Source*	*Secondary Source*
	service area, county, region and state			
	Illegitimate live births by zipcode, service area, county, region and state	Annually	Local or state health departments	
	Total live births by race by zipcode, service area, county, region and state	Annually	Local or state health departments	
	Fertility rate by county, region, state and nation	Annually	Local or state health departments	
	Mortality Data:			
	Number of deaths by zipcode, service area, and county For all causes By major causes of death	Annually	Local or state health departments	HSA
	Crude Death Rates:			
	(Deaths per 100,000 population) by service area, county, region, state and nation For all causes By major causes of death	Annually	Local or state health departments	HSA
	Number of infant deaths by zipcode, service area and county	Annually	Same as above	Same as above
	Infant Death Rates:			
	By zipcode, service area, county, region, state and nation Infant death rate (deaths < 1 year/1,000 live births) Perinatal death rate (fetal deaths and deaths < 7 days/fetal deaths and live births) Neonatal death rate (deaths < 28 days/1,000 live births)	Annually	Same as above	
	The leading causes of death by service area, county, region, state and nation	Annually/Biennially	Local or state health departments	HSA
	Selected communicable disease incidences (TB, VD, etc) by zipcode, service area, county, region and state Number of cases Rates/100,000	Annually	Same as above	State Health Dept.

Type of Data	*Basic Elements*	*Frequency of Collection*	*Primary Source*	*Secondary Source*
Service Area and Region Health Resource Inventory and Utilization Data:	*Short Term Acute Care Inpatient Resources:* Acute care bed complement by clinical service (OR, Ped, Adult M/S, Psych, etc) Total for service area By institution	Annually	Local hospital council or survey of individual facilities	State Health Facilities Commission (state plan)
	% occupancy by service by hospital	Annually	Same as above	
	Length of stay by service by hospital	Annually	Same as above	
	Total patient days used by the service area population (any hospital) by clinical service	Annually	HSA or local hospital council	State Health Planning and Development Agency (SHPDA)
	Total admissions for the service area population (any hospital) by clinical service	Annually	HSA or local hospital council	State Health Planning and Development Agency (SHPDA)
	Total service area patient day use rates by clinical service $\frac{\text{days of care}}{\text{1,000 population}}$	Annually	Hospital Planning Dept.	
	Service area population admission rates by clinical service $\frac{\text{admissions}}{\text{1,000 population}}$	Annually	Hospital Planning Dept.	
	Comparison of the patient day use rates by clinical service for individual zipcodes, the total service area, the region, Michigan and other states	Annually/ Biennially	Hospital Planning Dept.	
	Comparison of admission rates by clinical service for zipcodes, the service area, region, Michigan and other states	Annually/ Biennially	Hospital Planning Dept.	
	Local, regional, state and national five-year trends by clinical service	Triennially	Local hospital council	Local and national Blue Cross
	Occupancy		SHPDA	
	Length of stay		DHEW	
	Methods of payment		AHA	Commission on Professional & Hospital Activities (CPHA)
	Service Area *Ambulatory Care Resources:* (Hospital-based or free-standing)			
	Emergency Room Services ER classification by facility	Annually	HSA or regional EMS corporation	Local hospital council or survey of individual facilities

Type of Data	*Basic Elements*	*Frequency of Collection*	*Primary Source*	*Secondary Source*
	Number of ER visits by facility % ER visits admitted by facility			
	Zipcode patient origin data to determine ER service area	Annually	Sample survey by Hospital Planning Dept.	
	Outpatient Clinic Services: Clinics by type of facility Visits by clinic by facility Case load capacity by clinic by facility	Annually	HSA	Survey of individual facilities
	Zipcode patient origin data to determine outpatient clinic service area	Annually	Sample survey by Hospital Planning Dept.	
	Long-Term Care Resources:	Annually		
	Number and location of Skilled/basic nursing homes Homes for the aged (residential facilities)		State Health Facilities Commission (state plan) State Health Facilities Commission (state plan)	Survey of individual facilities Survey of individual facilities
	Skilled nursing beds and intermediate or basic beds:	Annually		HSA
	Total number for service area		State Health Facilities Commission (state plan)	
	Number by institution % occupancy by institution		Survey of individual facilities	Local hospital council
	Projected surplus or shortage of skilled/basic beds	Annually	State Health Facilities Commission/Hospital Planning Department	HSA
	Mental Health Resources:			
	Number and location of inpatient psychiatric facilities Long-term acute Short-term acute After-care facilities	Annually	Local mental health board	State Department of Mental Health (state plan)
	Number of beds and occupancy by facility Long-term acute Short-term acute	Annually	Local mental health board/State Dept. of Mental Health (state plan)	Survey of individual facilities
	Outpatient and crisis intervention services: Programs & facilities Case load capacity	Annually	Same as above	Same as above
	Substance Abuse Resources:			
	Inpatient Services: Total number of beds in service area Number of beds by facility	Annually	HSA	Survey of individual facilities/programs

Type of Data	*Basic Elements*	*Frequency of Collection*	*Primary Source*	*Secondary Source*
	% occupancy by facility Length of stay by facility			
	Outpatient Services: Number of programs/ facilities in service area Case load capacity of program/facility Visits by facility	Annually	Same as above	Same as above
	Manpower Resources:			
	Total number of MDs in service area	Annually	State licensing/ regulation body	State/local medical society
	Total number of DOs in service area			HSA Michigan Cooperative Health Information System Pharmaceutical firms Local hospital council
	Service area zipcode map of physician offices (primary office location for each physician)	Annually	Hospital Planning Dept.	
	Total number of dentists in service area and zipcode distribution	Annually	State licensing/ regulatory body	State/local dental societies Michigan Cooperative Health Information System HSA
	Total number of active RNs/LPNs in service area	Annually	State licensing/ regulatory body and	
	Total number inactive RNs/LPNs in service area		Michigan Cooperative Health Information System	HSA
	Total number of parapro-fessional or allied health personnel	Annually	Same as above	Same as above
	Local training programs	Annually	HSA	
	Regionalized Specialty Resources:			
	Neonatal intensive care services: Number and location of NICUs Total number of beds in service area Number beds by unit	Annually	HSA	Survey of individual facilities
	Admission by unit Patient days by unit % occupancy by unit	Annually	HSA	Survey of individual facilities
	A.L.O.S. by Unit Number deliveries in unit Number deliveries referred			

Type of Data	*Basic Elements*	*Frequency of Collection*	*Primary Source*	*Secondary Source*
	Burn Care Services: Number and location burn centers Number and location burn units Number and location burn programs	Annually	National Institute of Burn Medicine (NIBM)	Survey of individual facilities
	Radiation Therapy Units: Total number in service area Number by Institution	Annually	HSA	Local hospital council Survey of individual facilities
	Hemodialysis Units: Total acute and chronic units in service area Number acute and chronic units by institution		HSA	Local hospital council Survey of individual facilities
	Community Health Resources: Public Health Education Programs: Prenatal care Nutrition Family planning Chronic disease prevention others	Annually	Local health departments United Fund	Survey of individual agencies
	Home Health Agencies: Public/nonprofit Proprietary	Annually	HSA	United Fund Survey of individual agencies
	Public Health Clinics: VD TB Dental Medicaid screening Immunizations Mothers and infants others	Annually	Local health dept.	HSA Survey of individual agencies
III. Special Studies	Identification of specific service area needs/ problems	As appro-priate	Cooperative study by service area hospitals and local HSA	Hospital Planning Department Private consultant University Research Dept.
	Impact study concerning new developments in service area resources	Same as above	Hospital Planning Dept.	Private consultant
	Market research in connection with specific program or service	Same as above	Hospital Planning Dept.	Private consultant
	Financial feasibility study	Same as above	Accounting firm	

Source: Leonard Felgner, Chief Operating Officer, H.M.A., 210 Huron View, Ann Arbor, Mich. 48103. Reprinted by permission.

Part III

The Operational Planning Part of MBO

Chapter 6

How to Set Overall Hospital Annual Objectives

While strategic planning typically refers to long-range time frames, operational planning usually corresponds to the budget cycle. For most organizations this means the 12-month period making up their fiscal year, though for some institutions supported by public moneys it might mean a 24-month period.

The most common approach to begin the process of setting short-range objectives is a top management retreat of approximately two days (16 to 20 working hours). Participants in this retreat should include the CEO and all members of what is often called the administrative council or cabinet, together with representation (even if only token) from the medical staff and the board of trustees, for the same reasons we discussed earlier for their participation in the long-range planning process.

The retreat is an activity the aim of which is to come up with an overall plan or list of objectives and, where appropriate, supporting action steps to accomplish them. This list will be used as the basis for all the objectives at all other levels in the organization. While this list will appropriately be considered the "hospital's overall objectives," it is also emphatically considered the CEO's personal list of objectives, for it comprises the results he/she will commit to the board as custodian of the human, financial, physical, aesthetic, and informational resources of the institution.

The CEO must be personally present for this retreat. It is not an assignment to reasonably try to delegate to someone else. No one can do the CEO's management planning and management decision making for him or her.

By the same token, the CEO is not going to do all the work to achieve these results, so the presence of other top administrators is essential, in order that they be satisfied with the list as it is being prepared. Finally, administrative unanimity on these overall hospital objectives will not go very far unless they have the support of the board and the medical staff, so their nominal input at the very formulation stage will be helpful to keep the process from going "off the deep end" at the very beginning.

A simple definition of *objective* will help spell out a reasonable sequence of steps to arrive at such a list and will provide an outline of this chapter.

An objective can be defined as *the amount and direction of change from the present desired in a given period of time.*

Because you always wish to set realistic objectives, and what is realistic to achieve often depends on where you're starting from, it is necessary to look first at where you are now. Depending on that, a proposed objective might or might not be realistic; depending on that, one or another plan of action might be appropriate.

If you were talking about where you want to go or be in a physical sense only, it might be quite simple to state where you are—geography is readily apparent. But you are concerned here with the total welfare of the organization, and it is quite normal to have differences of opinion as to the current situation. Until some of these differences are reconciled, major assets and liabilities are listed, and some consensus as to your basic purpose is reached, you will not get very far trying to set objectives supported by all. You must start with a realistic analysis of the present, as considered in Chapter 5.

Objectives should be stated in such a way that "when we get there, we will know we are there." They will include, therefore:

- the objective area, or what it is you are trying to change
- an indicator of success, or way to measure change
- the specific amount of change desired in the time period ahead

It will usually be helpful to indicate which component unit or manager will be primarily responsible for the achievement of each objective. (We know coordination does not just happen by itself.) Component unit objectives can then be set to support institutional objectives. In some instances, these objectives will be stated exactly the same as for the hospital; other times they will simply express a contribution to the total result as appropriate for the one unit/department.

All objectives are then to be supported by *programs* or *action* steps planned to achieve the results. At times these are simply ongoing activities that might not even have to be recorded again on paper. But these activities are a means to the end results; they deal with *process* while objectives deal with *results*.

Participants in the retreat should now share with the group their recommended one-year objectives. As each person reads one, the discussion

Exhibit 6-1 First Draft of Annual Objectives

Key Result Area	*As Measured by*	*Present Level*	*Desired Level*

leader should enlist the aid of the group to help to rephrase it so each of the columns in Exhibit 6-1 can be completed.

Question: Now, develop objective statements on Exhibit 6-1. If you experience trouble figuring out what to put under "as measured by," refer back to the trend analysis for the ways to measure discussed in Chapter 5.

Exhibit 6-2 is an example of a completed list.

COMPLETENESS OF THE DRAFT

The exercise discussed in this chapter will result in a first draft of the annual objectives of your hospital. There are still a couple of things the group will want to do about the draft before adjourning. The first is to check its completeness.

The draft, after all, was put together from the limited offerings of all participants on a rather random basis. To check whether all the bases have been covered, these three approaches are suggested:

1. Review quickly the strong and weak points, as well as the trend analysis, to see if all the major items have been at least considered. This does not mean that all topics will be translated into objectives, but there should not be any that were overlooked inadvertently. Be

Exhibit 6-2 Sample Annual Objectives

Key Result Area	*Indicator*	*Present Level*	*Minimum*	*Desired Level Average*	*Maximum*
1. Productivity	a. FTEs per occupied bed	4.4	4.1	4.0	3.9
	b. Productive nursing hours per patient day				
	(1) Critical care	20.0	17.6	17.0	16.0
	(2) All other units	7.0	6.5	6.0	5.5
	c. No. of departments with completed standards of productivity	7/30	18/30	25/30	32/30
	d. FTEs per equivalent occupied bed	3.8	3.63	3.6	3.58
2. Fiscal Responsibility	a. No. of accounts receivable days (gross)	72.5	55	50	47
	b. No. of accounts receivable days (exclusive of Medicare and Medicaid)	75.5	68	62	58
	c. Credit balance days	5.6	2.2	1.82	1.5
	d. Active participation in Monotrend		by 7/1/81	by 5/1/81	by 3/1/81
	e. Excess of revenue over expenses (before adjustments)	$1.289 million	$1 million	$1.113 million	$1.12 million
	f. Profit margin (contrib: excess revenue as a percentage of gross patient revenue)	3.4%	2.5%	2.77%	2.79%
	g. Percent bad debt	5%	5%	4%	3%
	h. Revenue per equivalent patient day	$326	$382	$390	$398
	i. Expenses per patient day	$307	$360	$353	$346

3. JCAH Accreditation	a. Length of accreditation	1–2 years	2 years	2 years	2 years
	b. No. of compliance recommendations not adequately responded to	—	1	0	0
4. Inpatient Utilization	a. No. of patient days	100,282	95,933	100,000	105,000
	b. Occupancy (percent of staffed beds)	74.3%	75.4%	78.5%	82.5%
	c. No. of surgical hours	10,500	11,000	11,458	12,000
	d. Admissions	11,237	10,595	11,050	11,602
	e. No. of new physicians referring patients		3	4	6
5. Medical Staff	a. No. of communities served by physician outreach program	½	1	2	3
	b. No. of new young general surgeons admitted to staff	—	1	2	3
	c. Completion of physician surveys to determine level of satisfaction	—	80	100	120
	d. No. of physicians admitting over 10 patients per month	32	35	38	40
	e. Completion of reorganization of medical staff structure	Under discussion	Review of consulting corp. recommendations	Approval by medical staff	Implementation
6. Facilities Improvement	a. Completion of renovations of:		Old ICU Signage Cosmetic touch-up of patient areas Employee Cafe. Linear Acceleration Rehab Employees Locker	Minimum + near term parking and ER	Average + lab and facade of building north wing

Exhibit 6-2 continued

Key Result Area	*Indicator*	*Present Level*	*Minimum*	*Desired Level Average*	*Maximum*
	b. Long-range facilities plan	Consultant study	Report completed	Report accepted by board	Next year's action determined
	c. Medical office bldg.	Land-leased resolved Parking being discussed	Drawings completed; funding arranged by 7/1/81	Min. + construction begun	Average + construction begun by 9/1/81
7. Quality Care	a. No. of repeat deficiencies of established criteria	45%	45%	25%	0%
	b. No. of patient incidents (medical errors plus patient falls)	1916	2108	1916	1760
	c. Average waiting time for inpatient admissions		15 min.	12 min.	10 min.
	d. Nosocomial infection rate	4.4	4.1	3.9	3.5
	e. No. of incomplete charts	550	475	425	350
	f. No. of late operative reports	18–20	10	8	6
	g. No. of late histories and physicals	18–20	10	8	6
	h. Percent of patients with nursing care plan within 24 hours of admission	25%	66⅔%	75%	90%
	i. No. of depts. implementing appropriate quality assurance/control programs	7/34	26/34	30/34	34/34

8. Hospital Image	a. Percent of physicians evaluated overall care "1" or "2" on survey	—	75%	80%	85%
	b. Percent of patients who would not recommend the hospital to others on a survey	4–5%	4%	3%	2%
	c. Response rate for patient survey	10–18%	20%	25%	30%
	d. No. of press releases or human interest articles submitted to and used by Corp. Public Relations		8	10	12
	e. No. of new auxilians	25	30	40	50
	f. No. of job descriptions calling for auxilians	9	20	30	40
9. Management Contracts	a. Contract with ______	Contract maintained	Maintain contract	Maintain contract	Maintain contract
	b. Contract with ______	Contract maintained	Maintain contract	Maintain contract	Maintain contract
10. Outpatient Utilization	a. Total occasions of service including minor surgery in E.R.	7430	6907	7500	8000
	b. Integration of services into a coordinated outpatient program	Discussion stages	PT, OT, x-ray, lab, speech, EEG	Minimum + centralized outpatient admitting	Average + dialysis and radiation therapy
11. Human Resources	a. No. of EEOC complaints	4	3	2	1
	b. No. of late personnel evaluations per month	—	1	0	0
	c. No. of employee suggestions implemented	12	30	35	40
	d. Completion of compensation study	Grades determined	3/31/81	3/15/81	3/1/81

Exhibit 6-2 continued

Key Result Area	*Indicator*	*Present Level*	*Minimum*	*Desired Level Average*	*Maximum*
	e. No. of depts. showing some improvement in the attitude survey:				
	(1) job satisfaction		16/34	20/34	25/34
	(2) communication with depts.		20/34	25/34	28/34
	(3) participation in hospital decisions		20/34	25/34	28/34
	f. Percent of first level supervisors who work out personal development plans with their dept. head		50%	60%	70%
12. New Programs	a. No. of dept. directors generating innovative programs to impact on patient days		24/34	26/34	28/34
	b. New inpatient service		Feasibility study completed	Minimum + decision made	Average + plans completed to implement
	c. Conversion to new EDP in cooperation with Corp.	Under study	12/81	10/81	9/81
	d. Health screening program		Feasibility study	Minimum + decision made	Average + implementation

	e. Implementation of MBO	Training sessions	Goals negotiated for admin. and dept. heads	Minimum + evaluation against goals	Minimum + evaluation against goals
	f. Satisfaction with MBO by those using it		66⅔%	75%	80%
	g. Oncology satellite program which generates patient days		———	———	———
13. Education	a. Freshman enrollment in school of nursing for June 1981 and Jan. 1982	32	40	50	60
	b. No. of graduate nurses not passing the state board the first time	1	1	0	0
14. Retirement Home	a. Excess of revenue over expenses	−$50,000	0	$10,000	$15,000
	b. Occupancy rate	96.8%	96.8%	97.6%	97.6%
	c. JCAH accreditation	2 years	2 years	2 years	2 years
15. Shared Services	a. Cooperation with Corporate in centralizing the following services:		EDP, cash management and pur-chasing	Minimum + identify other candidates	Minimum + identify other candidates
	b. Development of formal plan for management contract and other shared services by:		11/81	10/81	9/81

sure, too, that objectives build upon your strong points as well as your weak points.

Take time now to review your draft of objectives against the earlier needs information. If anything important was left out, add it to the list.

2. Recall the use to be made of organizational objectives. There are two main uses: (1) they are to be used by the CEO to control the entire hospital, and (2) they are to be used by others as a guide (cue) in setting their supportive objectives. As a second way to check completeness of your draft, you should look over the list and ask:
   - Does the list include all the major results that the CEO will want to monitor regularly to see that the hospital is living up to its mission, and for which the CEO wishes to be held accountable?
   - Does the list include something into which at least the major departments can tie?

   Take time now to review your draft of objectives by asking the above two questions as a check on the use of the hospital's objectives. If anything important was omitted, add it to the list.
3. The CEO might have entered the discussion with a preconceived list of key results areas that he/she believes ought to be given high priority in the objectives list. (This was the recommended approach in an ongoing implementation of MBO in Chapter 3.) That list might have included such items as:
   - quality of care
   - support services
   - medical staff
   - new programs
   - financial stability
   - organization development
   - facilities and equipment utilization
   - outgoing operations
   - community and public relations
   - long-range planning

   Take time for the CEO to check his/her list of major areas of concern against your first draft. If anything important was left out, add it to the list.

PRIORITIZING THE DRAFT

The last advice the CEO probably wants to get from the group before adjourning is to rearrange the objectives on the list in terms of priorities.

The assumption ought to be that the list is put together in the light of information available today, and it is intended that all objectives on the list be accomplished. However, given the uncertainties of the future, no matter how well the group tries, it could be necessary to pare the list later on. So it is often helpful at this time to designate the relative priority of each objective.

A simple device for doing this is to score each objective on the list according to these three degrees of importance:

1. signifies important and essential
2. signifies important and necessary
3. signifies important, but if something has to go, this is it

Next, the "score" given each objective is summed and the objectives are ranked in importance, lowest score indicating highest priority.

Take time to prioritize the objectives on your list by assigning a score of 1 to 3 to each and adding the scores.

Review by CEO

At this point you have in hand a list of your hospital's highest priority short-range objectives in draft form. The emphasis until now has been on participation by all key members of your group in developing this list. The belief is that this process builds support for the hospital's objectives on the part of those who will have most of the work in accomplishing them.

But in a very real sense, these objectives are the objectives of the CEO, who is to be held accountable for their accomplishment. If they are or are not achieved, it is the CEO who must answer. This personal responsibility would seem to demand that the CEO have the final say about what goes on this list of organizational objectives.

Suggestions are fine, but they must not turn the manager into a rubber stamp. Because the group is satisfied with them does not mean they necessarily meet other requirements, such as the demands of higher authority or the board. The CEO should, therefore, take the draft, sleep on it, reconsider the list later, modify it as he/she wishes to be accountable for it, and negotiate with the board.

SUMMARY

This chapter has presented a process that can be utilized by the CEO of the hospital to engage the assistance of a key group of advisers to accomplish two things: an analysis of where the hospital is at a point in time and the drafting of a list of annual (operational) objectives for the hospital. Both stages are done using measurable items of information. It should be noted that this same model applies to formulation of objectives by subunits or departments within the hospital. The next chapter will move the process down the organization to individual managers.

NOTES

1. Peter F. Drucker, *Management* (New York: Harper & Row, 1974), p. 438.

Chapter 7

How to Set Objectives with Individual Managers

Until now we have been looking at MBO from the point of view of the entire hospital or subunit (division or department). The purpose of this chapter is to provide answers to the questions that individual managers have as they start out with the new system of management; namely, "What steps are involved? How do I go about getting the advantages that have been pointed out?"

BASIC ASSUMPTIONS

We should start our discussion of how MBO works by stating a few of the basic assumptions leading to the development of the system we know today. They are:

- Groups that are allowed to do their own planning are generally more effective than those given preset plans.
- Individuals who are systematically encouraged and assisted in setting their own levels of achievement do significantly better than those who are not.
- Groups and individuals perform better and reach planned objectives more quickly when they are provided on a timely basis with reliable and objective information on their progress.
- Use of carefully structured rewards will provide motivation for improvement at all levels of performance.
- Professionals within an organization can do an excellent job as measured by the standards of their own fields but still fail to contribute to the achievement of overall objectives.

OPERATIONAL DEFINITION OF MBO

To begin to build a bridge between these assumptions and the skills that must be acquired, consider this operational definition of MBO:

> MBO is a continual process whereby superior and subordinate managers periodically identify their common objectives, define individuals' major areas of responsibility in terms of results expected of them, and use these agreed-upon measures as guides for operating each department and for assessing the contributions of each manager to the work of the entire organization.

Of course, there is nothing new in this. MBO includes such familiar tools as delineation of responsibilities, delegation of power, setting of objectives, control devices, standards of performance, and evaluation of results. But this only points out MBO's greatest attraction: its simplicity. It requires work, but the kind of work that everyone can understand.

There are six major ideas contained in this definition. An examination of these key elements will help you be prepared for your role.

1. Mutual Agreement. Superior and subordinate managers will be sitting down in matched pairs to work out agreement on priorities. You might have a mental picture, then, in all that follows, of yourself in a private meeting with another level of management. The purpose of the meeting is to work out an agreement participatively. That is, the agreement should be the result of two-way communications, not the thinking of only one party.

Perhaps the word that best describes the type of two-way communication intended in these meetings is "negotiation." A leading figure in labor negotiations explains that too often these two-way communication sessions fail because the participants enter the discussion with the attitude that they are engaged in a battle, or at least a game.[1] The name of the game seems to be "stomp the other guy into the ground! He loses—you win. That's a successful negotiation!"

Of course, experience proves that any contract or "agreement" arrived at in that manner would soon be ruined in the administration phase. The losing party will find many ways to "spike" the contract as time goes by. The best situation is the one in which both come away feeling that the terms of the agreement are satisfactory and realistic.

The agreement in this first element of our definition is one marked by honest discussion. But such emphasis on participation ought not to be interpreted as meaning there can be no tough bargaining or as meaning the subordinate has the only say in the content of the agreement.

After the discussion is over, the results should be considered as a *commitment*. Once the terms have been agreed upon they should be considered as a mutual promise, a managerial contract, so to speak (not a legal document). Superiors promise their subordinates that if the latter achieve the agreed-upon objectives, they must be judged as having done a satisfactory job and must be treated accordingly. Likewise, subordinates promise their superiors that if the former do *not* achieve the present objectives, (and there are no extenuating circumstances to explain why not), they have failed to perform adequately and should be treated accordingly.

This mutual agreement, which through a process of negotiation becomes a commitment on the part of both persons, underlies all the rest.

2. Common Objectives First. What is the content of the mutual agreement? The common objectives of the hospital or department must be the first area of discussion and agreement. Before you can begin to discuss your own work, you must have a clear understanding of, and commitment to, the common objectives of the organization.

The agreement on common objectives should be more of a mutual acceptance and commitment than a matter of bargaining because, it is assumed, common objectives will have been determined long before this meeting. But the agreement is important because people are more easily reconciled to work expected of them if they are shown how it fits into the total picture. In addition, it is easier to make consistent decisions when there is an adequate frame of reference against which to measure smaller problems.

Commitment to objectives, then, should start at the top and work down. There can and should be input from the bottom up to help top management know what the overall hospital objectives should be, as was noted in Chapter 3. But now we are trying to understand what a manager at any level should do in using MBO. This second element in our definition is reminding us that the organization is probably structured according to the bureaucratic pyramid sketched briefly in Figure 7-1.

The role of each manager in such a structure is to serve as a "linking pin."[2] That is, your role is to look up, take the direction set by your superior, and interpret it for your own subordinates when you negotiate with them. In Figure 7-1, for example, the assistant administrator of support services, as part of top management, has a share in working with the CEO in identifying overall hospital objectives. Because of a share in setting these goals, he/she is committed to do what is necessary in support services to achieve them and, therefore, sees to it that objectives are set at this level that will support the hospital's objectives. Then the assistant administrator works with division managers to set objectives at their level

Figure 7-1 "Linking Pin" Organizational Concept

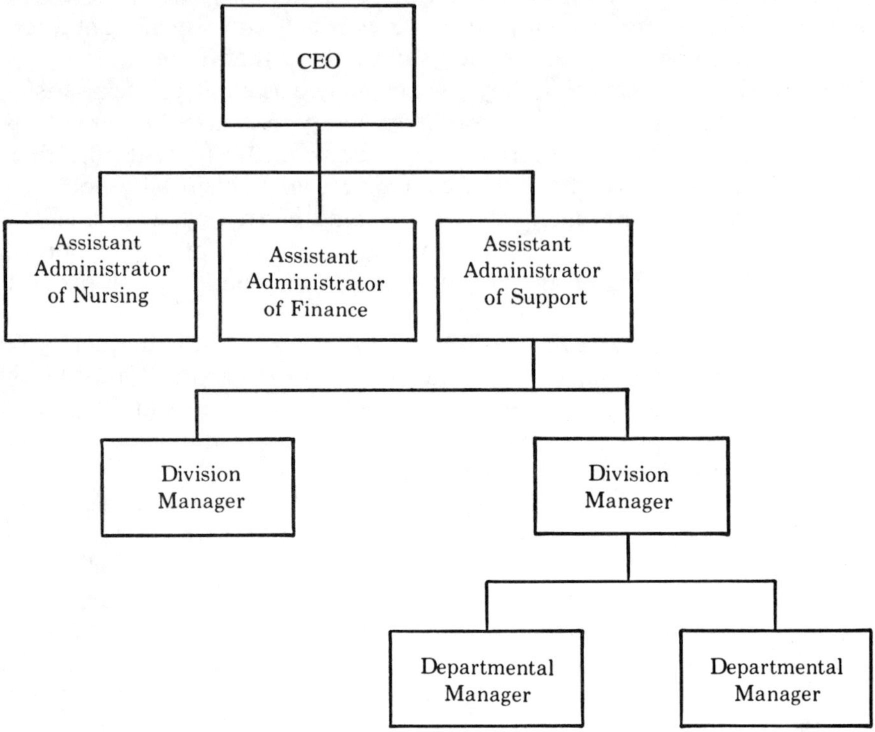

in such a way that these tie into support service objectives, thus completing the link. The same thing is repeated by the division managers with their department managers, and so on through the entire organization. Overlapping links form a chain. This is how the whole organization becomes integrated vertically into one chain or system of objectives.

Once there is agreement (and commitment) on these common objectives, there is less likelihood that an individual will set objectives in a different direction. Quite the opposite. The common objectives set the stage for developing objectives at a subordinate level that make it possible to accomplish the common objectives. Subordinates, then, are to take their cue from the statement of common objectives. These become "the game plan," as it were, so individual members of the team can discern what is expected of them in turn.

The primary role in this step is, of course, the superiors'. It is their responsibility to communicate, explain, and if necessary defend the overall objectives. Subordinates cannot support objectives that are unknown, not understood, or thought to be incorrect or meaningless. This is not the first time for subordinates to learn about the common objectives. But this is a final opportunity to review them and their meaning in the context of the subordinates' duties.

3. Major Responsibilities (Key Result Areas). Once the team's objectives have been clarified or the game plan reviewed, it is time to focus on the contributions of the individual in helping achieve the overall objectives. The superior and subordinate next go over the particular duties assigned to the subordinate. They answer the questions: "What is my job? Why was I hired? What role do I play on this team?"

In this meeting, subordinates suggests what their major assignments are in meeting common objectives and receive the superiors' confirmation or amendments.

For the most part, these are general duties as defined in the subordinates' job description. Subjects that might also be covered in this step are (1) job areas not covered in a written guide, (2) the necessity for rewriting the job description because of expected changes in work assignments, or (3) the discovery that whole areas laid out in the description are not being done because of the press of other work.

You will recall from Chapter 1 that a common managerial need leading to the development of MBO was a lack of agreement that seems to develop between superior and subordinate on exactly what the subordinate's job is. It is for this reason that we deliberately try to build such agreement into the objective-setting interview, at least once a year. This can easily be accomplished by reference to the written job description. As a matter of fact, it is almost the only way to keep a valuable management tool, such as a job description, useful.

It has become fashionable in some circles to ridicule the job description, at least for managerial positions.[3] When they become "the property" of the staff person involved in preparing them, instead of a tool used by management, they deserve to be ridiculed. But a job description can be revitalized in the MBO interviews simply by being reviewed. It thereby becomes much more useful than the crash programs of revising job descriptions we seem to go through periodically.

4. Short-Term Individual Objectives. So far subordinates have answered the question "What is my job?" with the help of their superiors. Now they must determine, "How will we know that I am doing that job well?" The answer to this question is found in the subordinate's objectives: for each major responsibility accepted by the subordinate, short-term, specific objectives should be set. Typically, these major projects or improvements are expected to be completed within 12 months. Taken together they comprise the "performance budget," or plan, for the coming year. Some important aspects of these objectives are:

- They should flow from the position description.
- They should be consistent with, and take their cue from, overall hospital objectives.
- They must be measurable, a requirement that encompasses the development of appropriate yardsticks to measure progress, or standards of performance.
- They must be challenging enough to provide motivation and a feeling of real accomplishment.
- They must be attainable and reasonably within the areas of influence of the individual.
- The total number of targets should be limited initially. After a while managers can handle more objectives effectively.
- Priorities should be assigned, even if only informally, to reach agreement on rank of importance whenever difficulties arise regarding allocation of resources.

If the objectives meet the above requirements, they will serve their function well: to let both superiors and subordinates know when performance is satisfactory; to let them know the subordinates have arrived at where they set out to go.

Likewise your work objectives must be stated so clearly that when you get there you will know you have arrived. Therefore, statements of objectives should be accepted only if they are that precise or measurable. All this emphasis on measurability has led some critics to decry MBO as "mechanistic," "overly quantifiable," "inhuman," and so forth. Sometimes those charges are deserved (when MBO is not practiced properly), but the need for specificity should not be equated with a demand for numbers. We will see when we start working out detailed examples that there are many ways to measure, and numerical counting is only one way. Sometimes we are more interested in the quality of a result than its quantity.

The real point here is that a helpful objective must do more than point you in a direction. It must spell out how far you wish to go in that direction. A football team doesn't score any points for moving the ball in a northerly direction: the ball must go the full 100 yards in that direction within certain time limits and within certain lateral boundaries, too. An objective then, as described earlier, is the *direction and degree (amount) of change from the present desired within a specified period of time.*

If that is so, then statements we sometimes call "objectives" will be seen as not fitting the definition. For example, there is probably not a hospital manager alive who has not been told somewhere along the line, "we have only one objective really: to provide the highest quality patient care possible." As it stands, that statement is a poor objective because it doesn't tell us when we have achieved the result we are after, when we have arrived. It points in a direction, but does not say how much progress in that direction is acceptable as realistic in a given time span. It is a poor objective statement because it does not serve the function of an objective, not because anyone is against high quality patient care! That would be the same as being against motherhood, the flag, and the Fourth of July. But we should get the motherhood out of our objectives.

Is there a place for motherhood statements? Of course. We recommended in the previous chapters that top management provide employees with an opportunity to understand the hospital's basic purpose in a statement of its mission, or its credo. It is good to be dedicated to these things. They simply do not belong in objectives.

5. Use of Performance Budget. The term *performance budget* was used in the preceding section to describe the sum total of a person's objectives. This was deliberate. It is not done to draw attention to finances, which is probably what comes to mind at the sight of the word *budget,* but to suggest the use to be made of the list of objectives. Once individuals' objectives are agreed upon and reduced to writing, they have a plan for the next period of operations. But we said MBO is more than planning: it is a total system of management. So the objectives must serve as more than a plan.

The word *budget* suggests how the objectives are to be used. The preparation of a capital budget or an expense budget is just the beginning. It must then be used as a guide during the period covered, and it is used as a means of evaluating fiscal control when the period is over. This is the same pattern that should apply to the performance budget, or list of objectives. During the period covered, it should be used as a guide for making decisions and monitoring progress. If it has been prepared well, it will include checkpoints along the way to see if progress is satisfactory to that point. There will be stated intervals of time for taking a reading to see if ongoing performance is at a satisfactory level.

All this means that the objectives that have been agreed upon must be reduced to writing and referred to continuously as a means of controlling actions. You, as subordinate, should refer to this written instrument daily for guidance in allocating time and energy and for distribution of the resources available. Ultimately, you should do nothing that is not connected somehow with the agreed-upon list of objectives because, by definition, they constitute what you and your superior agreed was your workload.

It is here that MBO can be seen as a tool for the development of subordinate supervisors. By learning to refer to their lists of objectives and what is learned to be the objectives of others, managers learn to make decisions rather than wait for higher authority to say what to do. The help of the administrative superior has already been given in developing the objectives. After that, the subordinates should learn to "stand on their own two feet" by answering questions and solving problems using the norms expressed in their objectives. This serves to decentralize decision making in an organization very rapidly, as managers learn to monitor their own progress.

Superior managers also benefit because as subordinates are better able to handle their affairs, more time is available for superiors to do their own work. They are no longer required to exercise close supervision and can go on to other important work.

6. Basis of Formal Evaluation. If all year long managers monitor performance against the agreed-upon list of objectives, it follows that at the end of the year's operations, these same objectives should be used as the basis of any formal evaluation made by the administrative superior. The objectives provide the standards that are used to judge performance of the subordinate.

This use of objectives and the standards of performance they include have led many to define MBO as a "new method of performance appraisal." Experience shows, however, that when this is the major understanding of MBO (when it is seen as primarily a method of evaluation, or when it is stressed as a means of judging people or as a control mechanism), there are minimal results. Nobody likes to go before a judge, so as a rule there is resentment toward a system perceived primarily as a tool for being judged. On the other hand, when people appreciate all the other uses and benefits, they usually accept that the logical conclusion is to use the same standards as a way of judging satisfaction with what has been done or not done.

So this part of the definition of MBO and how it works is really saying two things:

1. There should be a formal evaluation of performance from time to time.
2. The basis of that evaluation should be one's own objectives.

Exhibit 7-1 Typical Trait Approach to Appraisal

PERFORMANCE EVALUATION							
	Superior	*Excellent*	*Very Good*	*Good*	*Fair*	*Poor*	*Unsatis-factory*
Ability							
Loyalty							
Initiative							
Cooperation							
_______							
_______							

Managers have committed themselves to apply all their resources toward a set of objectives, and an evaluation of their accomplishments should be based on these agreed-upon objectives, not on some other less meaningful set of criteria. These managers have literally staked their careers on achieving these objectives, insofar as they are able to control or influence the outcome, and they should be assessed on that basis. Chapter 17 is devoted to this subject of appraisal.

Most organizations are still using subjective methods of evaluating performance and will benefit from this aspect of MBO, if introduced properly. The typical appraisal form looks something like Exhibit 7-1. It is usually called a *performance* evaluation form, but the items listed for evaluation are basically personality traits: characteristics that, it is hoped, are found in all good employees. The difficulty is that even when there is an attempt at defining these terms, the only way to rank a person using them is by subjective judgment. Especially when the form uses the columnar approach (as shown in Exhibit 7-1), asking for a check in the appropriate box—that in itself is calling for a subjective judgment.

These subjective judgments are what have led most employees to resent the whole appraisal idea: they go before a supervisor who presumes to play God with their future by making evaluations on the basis of some sort of assumed superior knowledge, rather than on the basis of any demonstrable facts. Employees under such a system have little chance of receiving any real help. Either they have pleased the superior, who simply marks "performance" satisfactory, or they are not "in" with the superior, who proceeds to scold or demand unrealistic changes in personality without ever constructively showing the connection between such demands and actual job performance.

Because it is so difficult to justify a ranking—any ranking—using the approach in Exhibit 7-1, most superiors fail to make a convincing explanation, and most subordinates do not listen to the poor one that is given. Result? Little communication takes place. The upshot of the whole encounter is that raw nerves have been exposed; a piece of paper is signed and sent to "document" the subordinate's worth to the organization.

What has happened is that a *means* has become an *end* in itself. What should be discussed as tools to do a job (attitudes, skills, and traits) have been made the end-all and be-all of the evaluation because they are the items listed on the form. The subordinate does not understand why these highly personal characteristics are any concern of the superior and usually resists discussing them. (If you were not convinced it were any of your superior's business, you would prefer to choose your own analyst, if indeed you needed one!)

It is our opinion that hospitals are trapped in this situation. Some time ago, as business organizations grew more complex with more varieties of employees requiring some kind of centralized personnel administration, it seemed appropriate to "measure" their performance by some set of standard criteria, which could then be used for comparative purposes when it came to salary considerations, promotions, and the like. But how does one start such a system? Well, why not find out how they do it in the military, where reviews have been done for a long time? Of course, what might have made sense in an army, where discipline and rules and forming of a million copies of the same type performer might be appropriate, is not appropriate for business. Oh, it might serve a valid purpose during what is usually called the probationary period, when we find out if employees have certain basic working habits. We do want them to have ability, to show initiative, to be cooperative, to have loyalty, to be neat and clean, to come to work on time, and so on. But after they demonstrate that they have these characteristics, maybe we need not still be checking years later to see if they still have them!

This seems to be especially true when it comes to evaluating various types of managers. Again, where the Exhibit 7-1 approach is used, it is probably out of desperation. Casting about for an evaluation tool, the form used for hourly employees was handy—so it was turned into a form for supervisors as well. Copying or pirating to save time proved ineffective.

In recent years the weaknesses of the personality trait approach have become apparent to some groups working within various specialty areas.

They have been encouraged by their professional and paraprofessional associations to improve performance appraisal. Dieticians, housekeeping supervisors, and nurses, for example, have been working within their own professional organizations to devise better criteria for measuring performance. These have ranged from better definitions of the scale used (superior, excellent, etc.) to better definitions of the traits being ranked (job knowledge, initiative, etc.) to the incident approach, asking for essay-type descriptions of behavior to illustrate desirable or undesirable performance.

These types of forms probably make it easier for superiors to make a judgment; indeed, they often put words in their mouths in trying to capture what a subordinate does or does not do. But they ignore the issue of getting a preagreement from subordinates that these descriptions are in fact the kind of performance to which they originally committed themselves. Only an approach such as MBO gets the superior and subordinate to agree in advance on the criteria to be used to judge performance. And when this is done on an individual basis, as we have been stressing, then the real message comes through—that is, that subordinates are being appraised not to find out if they conform to some hypothetical ideal, but to find out if they are living up to legitimate commitments. The interest in evaluation is not in *who they are,* but in *what they achieve.* The competition is not against other employees to get a promotion, but against the challenge set in advance as a description of satisfactory performance. Viewed this way, the appraisal step is seen as the logical conclusion of the entire system.

HOW TO GET STARTED

Logical questions at this point might be, "Where do I start? How do I begin?" To implement the face-to-face idea exchange requires only four basic steps (even if the entire hospital is not going to formally use MBO as a system of management).

1. Clarify your working organization chart. Sketch out a chart showing only yourself and those managers reporting directly to you. For those managers, make a note of what responsibilities you feel they should have and especially which of the total hospital or unit objectives each one is most responsible for achieving. Also note any pending changes in division of authority.

   This is a necessary preliminary step you accomplish in private. For that very reason, it is also one that is easy to dismiss as a waste of time. There seems to be a tendency for busy managers to devote little time to such private work, yet experience shows that this kind of personal preparation is what keeps managers in charge of interviews when they take place, rather than their simply reacting to what subordinates submit.

We saw above that objectives flow from a discussion of a person's major duties. This step is your opportunity to reflect on what you believe your people's major duties are, and this is essential if MBO is to pinpoint that for which each person is to be held accountable. (We will elaborate on this further in the next chapter.)

2. Review the past performance record of each key subordinate. You cannot do an intelligent job of setting performance standards, or even assigning work responsibilities, unless you first take stock of your subordinates. This means examining prior performance reviews, salary progress, and career mobility, and possibly checking personnel department records or talking to a person's previous supervisor.

   You are trying to build a strong team. To do so you must know the strong and weak points of team members and then set objectives and standards of performance accordingly. This is the management function of organizing.

   This second preliminary step is essential if the interviews to follow are to set realistic objectives for each individual. The belief here is that different individuals, even with the same title (two head nurses), might have different objectives because of their different backgrounds, different capabilities, different surrounding circumstances. Notice then that MBO is not the purely mechanistic or mathematical model it is sometimes made out to be. It really is very human and individualistic when done well.

3. Hold the one-on-one negotiation meetings. Preparation is extremely important here. Subordinates must be given adequate notice of the meeting and convinced of its importance, and thus be willing to put significant time into preparing work objectives as they see them. Give each person a copy of your objectives so that you have something to tie you together.

   In a similar manner, you should be prepared to discuss what you see as each one's objectives, but be sure you maintain an open mind. This is the preparation needed by both of you. If there is to be true negotiation, you must each enter the discussion with a tentative idea of what you think appropriate for the other individual, as a starting point for the conversation. Of course, this starting point should be arrived at by some serious consideration on your part. There should be reasons for your tentative position. The better you are able to explain your reasons, the more likely the negotiating will proceed amicably. It is usually when one of the parties has done no serious reflecting that negotiations break down. Either the subordinate gives in, or the superior relies on positional authority to make decisions.

Some managers will prefer to have a copy of the subordinate's draft objectives to assist in preparation for this meeting. This can be very helpful. It also serves to reinforce the participative nature of setting objectives, since the subordinate is the one being asked to prepare the first draft. The danger is that the manager might simply take the written draft, make notes on it of what is liked or disliked, and return it to the subordinate with no face-to-face meeting. *This would be a serious mistake. You cannot negotiate objectives by memo.* The heart of MBO, what gives it real meaning, is the team building that can take place, the opportunity to learn each other's approach to getting the job done, the sincere mutual support that can be felt only in face-to-face discussion. No manager really wants to be involved in more meetings, but the MBO meetings should not be the ones to be cut off.

By couching an objective in poorly stated terms, a subordinate can receive a negative response from a supervisor when a favorable reaction is expected. The head of the anesthesia department might, for instance, state an objective as "the employment of an additional aide to assist with certain duties." Put this way, the objective is likely to receive a cold shoulder from a cost-conscious, budget-minded CEO. Through discussion, this CEO might learn that professionals are often used for sterilizing equipment or other nonprofessional chores. As a result they are not available for more surgical procedures. Another aide would free-up the professionals for more efficient utilization of the operating room. Presented with this information, the objective would quickly win approval because the objective sought now is not additional staff, but additional service and revenue. Additional people ought not be objectives in themselves, but means to some desirable objectives.

Before closing the meeting, offer your assistance: "What can I do to help you accomplish your objectives? What can I stop doing to help you achieve your objectives?" If subordinates' objectives spring from yours, as they should, if you have delegated a portion of your authority, then helping them achieve these objectives contributes to the attainment of your own. In the final analysis, you are measured by how well your people reach their objectives, so you are anxious to be helpful.

When agreement is reached on all this, put the statement in writing; both you and your subordinate keep a copy for future reference (daily).

4. Review your subordinates' performance budgets with them periodically. No plan is worth more than the follow-up attention it receives. Further, objectives should not be straitjackets that prevent freedom of movement as time passes. There must be opportunity to modify objectives according to changing circumstances—provided the change is made bilaterally, just as was the original objective. Therefore, you should check regularly to see:

   - that you are keeping to your commitment to assist your subordinate in attaining objectives
   - that progress is being made according to the standards of performance agreed upon
   - whether objectives need to be changed

   These can be done when you review the periodic report you will want to receive—perhaps monthly, perhaps less often. At a minimum you will wish to establish a regular routine for quarterly reexamination of the list of objectives.

SUMMARY

This chapter has attempted to set forth an operational definition of how MBO works from the point of view of the individual manager. No matter what level of responsibility you hold, you are called upon to meet individually with key subordinates (supervisors) and work out with them mutually agreeable objectives to support objectives at higher levels in the hospital. You serve as the linking pin in the organization, helping those you manage to take their cue from hospital or departmental objectives and translate them into measurable and realistic results in fulfilling their own major responsibilities.

The need for adequate time to prepare and for skillful exchange of ideas has been emphasized. The appraisal aspect of MBO should be seen as the logical conclusion of the system, as a freely accepted self-monitoring device, not as an authoritarian control mechanism or as the main reason for having MBO.

This chapter has focused primarily on process. Next we must move to content and form of objectives.

NOTES

1. Gerald I. Nierenberg, *The Art of Negotiating* (New York: Hawthorn, 1968).
2. Rensis Likert, *New Patterns of Management* (New York: McGraw-Hill, 1961).
3. Robert Townsend, *Up the Organization* (New York: Knopf Publishing Co., 1970).

Chapter 8

How to Identify Key Result Areas

Thus far we have reviewed the process of developing overall organizational objectives (hospital or department) and the face-to-face objective-setting and monitoring by matched pairs of managers. With this overview of how the system operates at the group or pair level, each manager ought to be ready to study and practice setting objectives as an individual.

Natural questions of any manager beginning to implement the system are: "Where do I begin?" "What steps are involved?" Stated simply, they are:

1. Define your key result areas (KRAs).
2. Determine how to measure success in each area.
3. Take stock of your present performance in each area, using the measurement indicators chosen.
4. Prepare a draft of the level of performance to which you are ready to commit yourself.
5. Negotiate all the above with your immediate administrative superior.
6. Monitor progress as the weeks go by.
7. Review performance with your superior at least quarterly.
8. Summarize the year's results at the end of the year in a review session with your superior as the basis for starting the entire cycle over again the following year.

The purpose of this chapter is to review the mechanics of the first of these steps, the development of your KRAs.

WHAT IS A KEY RESULT AREA?

A prevailing attitude among many persons who hesitate or refuse to commit themselves to objectives is the belief, "You can't measure my work." You hear this especially from those who deal with intangibles, with values, and with services, as opposed to those whose jobs involve more immediately visible results (manufactured items, dollars, buildings, etc.)

It is probably more true to say that some jobs are more difficult to measure than others, but not impossible, and that that difficulty is reduced greatly when we realize that it is difficult to measure *any* job in its entirety. We shouldn't be trying to measure the *whole* job of a nurse, a business office manager, or an executive housekeeper, any more than that of a personnel manager, an engineer, a public relations director, the legal counsel, or others.

We don't measure the whole job; we break it down into its component parts. We itemize the separate responsibilities or duties that the job entails. Those discrete parts of the job we call key result areas. They are not objectives, but they are areas of concern, which we will turn into objectives. They will become objectives when we determine how to measure them and add a precise level of accomplishment or change. But before we measure, we have to know what we are trying to measure. A KRA, then, is the answer to the questions, "What is it I am trying to measure? What are the things for which I am accountable? What are the major components of my job?" If I'm like most people, I will probably find I perform some of my responsibilities in an outstanding manner; others I do rather well; some I am about average in; still others I'd just as soon hide under the carpet. This means that some will not need any measurable improvement, while others will require varying degrees of improvement. Only if I begin identifying these different areas will I then be able to make some commitments as to how much improvement I ought to be making in each part of my job, since I'm not doing the whole job at a uniform level of excellence.

HOW TO FIND KRAs

What you list as your KRAs ought to be stated in output terms. We must remember not to fall into the activity trap or the input trap discussed in Chapter 1.

Question: How did we define an input (as opposed to an output)?
Answer:

You should have recalled that an input is an asset, a resource, something needed to do your work, a tool, a means as opposed to an end.

Question: How did we define an activity (as opposed to an output)?
Answer:

You should have recalled that an activity is some expenditure of energy, a program, something you do as opposed to something you make happen (create), another means as opposed to an end.

The important thing in searching for KRAs, then, in all that follows here, is to remember to state them in *results* terms, not in action terms. The use of *nouns,* rather than *verbs,* might be helpful in this regard. Verbs are action words and are difficult to measure. Nouns, however, have all kinds of properties and qualities—size, dimensions, scope, frequency, shape, and the like—which will be much easier to measure.

Your first source of KRAs is the organization chart. Look at the titles of the persons reporting to you. These are usually indicative of major areas of responsibility for which you are accountable. They are so major that you require someone else to take direct charge of them. These other persons have the day-to-day responsibility of getting results, but you still have to answer to your superior for what happens there.

For example, an assistant administrator of fiscal services might have an organizational chart as shown in Figure 8-1.

Question: Looking at Figure 8-1, what might be some of the KRAs for the assistant administrator?
Answer:

You should have noted at least the following:

- financial control/accounting
- payroll
- business office
- data processing

Question: Now referring to your own organization chart, are there any KRAs you could list as possibly belonging among your major accountabilities?

Figure 8-1 Fiscal Services Organization Chart

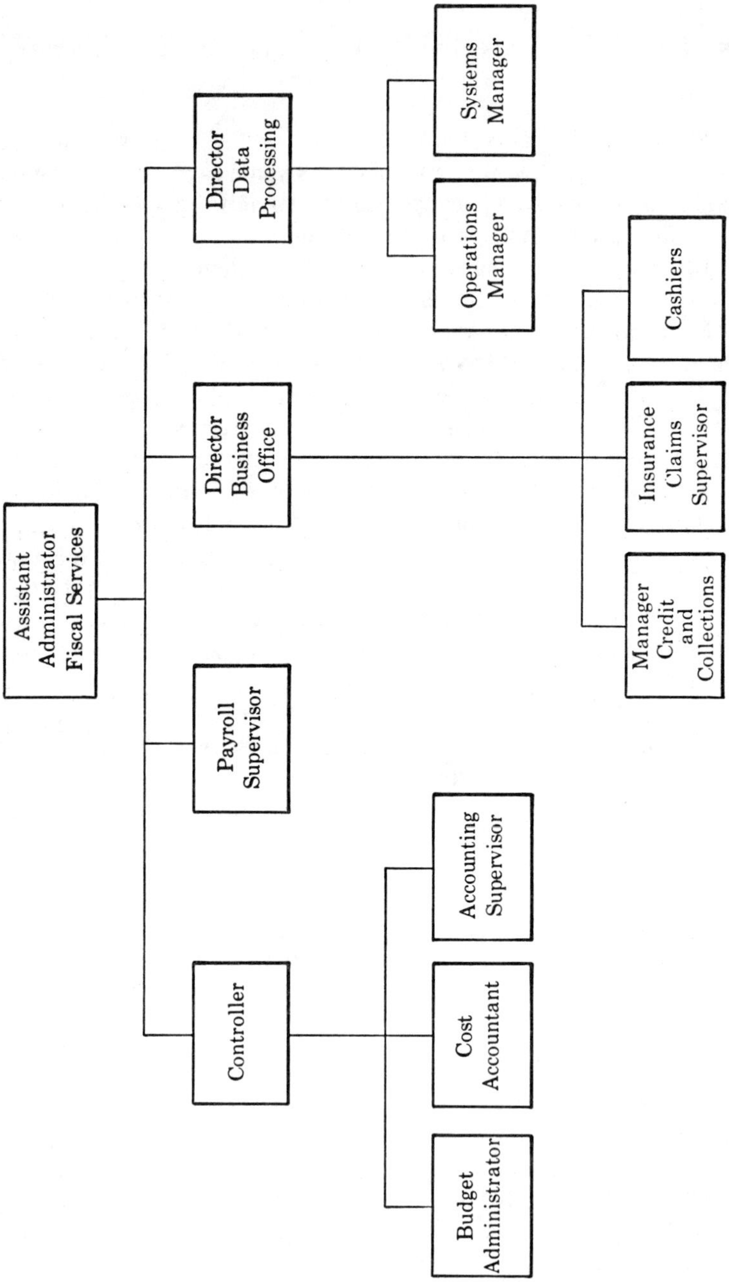

Answer:

A second source of KRAs is your job description. This document normally lists the major functions you are expected to perform. A *function* is defined as a "cluster of activities geared around a particular result." It is the *result* you are looking for here, not the activities or tasks. On an hourly person's job description we find a list of such tasks:

- sweeps the corridors daily
- takes dictation as required
- checks the locks twice a night

A manager's job description is usually expressed in broader terms (the function of clusters of tasks).

If your job description does not state those functions in results terms, if your major duties are too activity-oriented, you might have to ask yourself, "What results do I make happen when I do the action described in this paragraph?" All you're looking for is the *name* of it; do not worry about how much of it just yet.

A review of the job description for the assistant administrator whose organization chart we looked at above might reveal the following additional KRAs:

- financial obligations
- cash deposits
- staff recruitment
- staff development
- cost reductions
- space allocations
- budget preparation
- budget reporting

Now, suppose you are the controller. Your job description contains a paragraph to the effect that you are "responsible for maintaining sufficient cash balances in all accounts to meet all expenses in a timely manner."

Question: What would be the KRA for this function of the job?

Answer:

You should have said something like "cash flow" or "financial obligations."

Let's try another example. This time, suppose you are the personnel manager, and your description says you are "responsible for maintaining records for all employees."

Question: What would be the KRA for this function of the job?
Answer:

You should have identified the KRA as "employee record maintenance."

Again, suppose you are a medical records administrator, and your job description says you are "responsible for preparation of appropriate statistical summaries for administration and outside agencies."

Question: What would be the KRA for this function of the job?
Answer:

You should have said the KRA is "statistical summaries."

KRAs for a director of nurses might include:

- quality of care
- nursing audits
- budget administration
- staffing patterns
- patient safety
- physician relations
- staff development
- personnel administration

For a personnel manager, one would have to consider:

- recruiting/employment
- employee communication
- employee records

- training
- safety
- employee grievances
- salary administration
- personnel policy administration

Question: Now look at your own job description and come up with an itemized list of KRAs to add to those coming from the organization chart. (There may be some duplication.)

Answer:

The next source of KRAs is in the special programs, projects, committee assignments, and the like that have been delegated to you, even if they are not listed on your job description. The concept is that if you are *in charge of* such a program or committee, it probably should appear on your list of KRAs because you are chairing or managing it. (Simple membership on a committee or project would not be included on your list.)

Typical examples might be the safety committee, the grievance committee, a long-range planning committee, a disaster committee, the equal employment opportunity program, the environmental protection program, a committee to orient new employees, a space allocations task force, the data processing applications advisory committee, and so forth.

Question: Think of your special program/committee assignments and select a few to add to your KRAs.

Answer:

A final question to ask yourself in completing your list of KRAs, especially if you're having trouble so far, is "What have I made happen in the last few weeks/months on the job?" The answer to this question might suggest areas in which you are apparently causing results and could be a good way to get a handle on what you are accountable for producing in your job.

For example, perhaps you effected a management contract to administer a similar department as yours in a satellite facility, so you write "management contract." Or, perhaps you shepherded an application for additional beds through the local HSA, so you write "certificates of need." Or, you organized all the logistics for an open house during Hospital Week, to educate the public about your institution, so you write "community education."

A similar question might be, "What has my superior had occasion to ask me about in the past few weeks/months regarding my performance?" One CEO we know insists that all superiors have lists of pet things they fuss over with subordinates. This "fuss list" suggests some additional KRAs.

Question: Ask yourself these two questions and include on your list of KRAs the things you have made happen and/or the things your superior fusses with you about.

Answer:

As a check on the completeness of your list of KRAs coming from all four of the above sources and to start the process of ordering them in some sort of priority, take a look at the objectives of the organization (as shared with you by your administrative superior), and see if there are any on that list that suggest result areas to you because they identify things for which you are accountable or things to which you must obviously make a contribution.

For example, if one of the hospital's objectives is to reduce losses due to pilfering or break-in by 20 percent and you are a pharmacy manager, one of your KRAs should be related to that high priority area. Or, if there is an objective to reduce the number of late charges on patient bills by 50 percent and you are a lab supervisor, your KRAs should include this important topic. Should one of the support service division's objectives be to reduce by 25 percent the amount of overtime expenses, one of your KRAs should be identified accordingly.

Some lists of organizational objectives will have a column entitled "responsibility" to identify the particular departments or units expected to have supporting objectives. Some results will require supporting objectives from all managers, so such a responsibility column might say "all managers" as a reminder of that expectation.

Question: Beside each of the following sample organizational objectives, write an appropriate KRA for the persons whose titles are given:

Unit Objective	*Individual*	*KRA*
1. Review adequacy of existing physical facilities and re-examine long-range plans.	1a. Dir of Nurses	______
	1b. Controller	______
2. Establish automated patient records system.	2a. EDP manager	______
3. Review and revise the program for performance appraisal of managers.	3a. Personnel Mgr	______
	3b. Exec Housekeeper	______
	3c. Radiologist	______
4. Reduce expendable supplies expense by 13%.	4a. Bus Office Mgr	______
	4b. Head Nurse	______
	4c. Controller	______

Your answers should have looked something like this:

1a. Patient bed projections
1b. Financial projections
2a. Patient record system
3a. Management development
3b. Management development
3c. Management development
4a. Expendable supplies
4b. Expendable supplies
4c. Budget control

SHARED RESPONSIBILITIES

This last exercise points out the possibility of several individuals sharing responsibility for the same KRA. The entire system of MBO seeks to pinpoint responsibility by identifying who is responsible for what, but the real world is such that at times several persons must make a contribution in their separate domains if a single major result is to be achieved. The programs of action open to each will naturally be different, so people will not be getting in one another's way accomplishing the result. But without agreement first on a common end result and without recognition of the end result as a key one, chances for success are minimal.

As much as possible the KRAs should be the outputs that you *principally* control. You may not always *exclusively* control the result, however. Sometimes you only *influence* the outcome. For example, suppose you are in the controller's office, and you work in the area of getting budgets prepared for presentation to administration and/or the board of directors.

The various departments prepare their budgets and submit them to you, so really you do not author all these budgets, but you are expected to see that they are ready. Would it be valid to say that one of your areas of responsibility (KRAs) is "preparation of departmental budgets"?

Probably yes, even though you must rely on others and hence do not exclusively control the result. You should be able to influence them to prepare their budgets, probably with your assistance. This means you should list this as a KRA, and so should each of the department heads who also contribute to the same end result.

Similarly, if you were in the purchasing department and worked on preparing a catalog listing all the hospital's supply items, you would be jointly responsible for the KRA of "supply catalog" with the divisions that order the products and thus originate the list of items for the catalog.

THE ROLE OF STAFF PERSONS

This will be true in a very special manner for almost all staff or service offices, which will share responsibility for output with those whom they serve. Staff areas generally are more difficult to break down into their component parts, as we have been discussing in this chapter. These areas are where the real challenge for MBO lies today—and also where the greatest potential payoff lies.[1]

Staff functions generally fall into one or more of four basic areas:

1. Services—actual work performed for another department or office of the hospital (e.g., employing, printing, programming).
2. Advice—assistance in the form of counsel. Staff does not actually perform work but offers suggestions or recommendations to help solve a problem (e.g., legal counsel, personnel advice with relation to unions).
3. Control—supplying reports and other forms of data for the purposes of analysis, feedback, and so forth or requiring that certain procedures be followed in pursuit of hospital policies (e.g., salary administration, purchasing, accounting).
4. Research—conducting research efforts on present and anticipated areas of opportunity (e.g., research departments, library search, study groups, survey teams).

It might be, if you are a staff person, that you would simply list one or more of those four words among your KRAs.

Recognition of these areas of responsibility by staff persons and acceptance of being in part accountable for the results of these four kinds of staff contributions to the mission of the institution, despite the inability to totally control the results they bring about, will go a long way in causing increased communications between the staff individuals and others whom they are expected to advise or assist. This is perhaps the most significant way in which MBO contributes to horizontal (interdepartmental) communications, as opposed to the vertical (superior–subordinate) communicating that has been emphasized so far in this book.

Question: Now review your list of KRAs to date and see if you have included also those areas where you share responsibility for the outcome with someone else. Add to your list to include such joint accountabilities.

Answer:

SUMMARY

The place for an individual to begin in preparing objectives is the development of a list of KRAs. These are the principal duties, responsibilities, or component parts of the job. They are the areas for which the individual is to be held accountable. Taken together they answer the questions, "What is my job? What are the areas in which I am expected to make a contribution to the unit of which I am a member?"

NOTES

1. George Odiorne, "Management by Objectives: The Current State of the Art", unpublished monograph.

Chapter 9

How to Write Objectives

You have broken your job down into its component parts (KRAs), and you are ready to turn those responsibilities into objectives. You have decided that for which you are accountable. Now you want to know whether you are fulfilling those accountabilities in a satisfactory manner. You are going to want to determine this for yourself and then bring the results of your thinking to a negotiation session with your administrative superior to be sure you are in agreement.

THE SIMPLEST (SIMPLISTIC) APPROACH

There are as many suggested ways of writing objectives on paper (to capture the meeting of the minds you seek between matched pairs when they meet to negotiate objectives) as there are consultants in the field. The comments made here are based not on any presumed or claimed position of having the "best" or the "right" approach, but on the basis of demonstrated effectiveness.

About the simplest approach is that advocated by those who like to use the KISS principle (Keep It Short and Simple). They advocate using one short and simple formula for stating any objective. All you have to do is learn the formula, taking note of its essential parts, and crank out objective statements by simply filling in the appropriate blanks. The magic formula goes something like this:

To	*verb*	*noun*	by	*date*	at	*cost.*
	1	2		3		4

All that is required for an objective statement by this method is to fill in the four blank lines with the designated type of word. The first need is a verb, an action word, because objectives do not happen by themselves.

Then you need a noun, or the end result you are trying to accomplish. Third, you need a date because every objective should have a time element, or nothing is likely to happen. And finally, every objective has its price, so you should include a cost consideration, usually expressed in dollars, labor hours, or some resource expended to achieve the objective.[1]

Here are some examples of objective statements arrived at by simply providing the information for the four blanks in the formula:

- To *prepare* a long range *plan* for the hospital by *July 1* at a cost of *$10,000.*
- To *revise* the employee *handbook* by *September 1* at a cost of *$2,000.*
- To *purchase* three *typewriters* for our department by the start of the *quarter* at a cost of *$570* each.
- To *develop* a *training program* for new foremen for presentation to the maintenance manager by *Feb. 15* at a cost of *230 labor hours.*

Question: Critically evaluate any one of the above objective statements. Determine whether the one you select serves the function of an objective as discussed in previous chapters; that is, does it describe the job done in a satisfactory manner? Does it indicate the direction and degree of change from the present?

Answer:

No matter which of the above objective statements you chose, you should have noted that the statement, as it stands, does not have enough information to judge whether the job was done in a satisfactory manner when the date arrived. The main problem is that the statement only describes a resource to be acquired or a task to be performed; a plan is to be prepared; a handbook is to be revised; a program is to be developed. There is nothing in any of the statements that can help in determining whether the plan prepared is of any value, whether the handbook as revised does what it should, whether the program developed meets the needs.

Some will argue that all those things are taken for granted, that upon completion of a plan, a handbook, or a program, anyone can tell whether it was successful. We respectfully disagree and suggest that this is why we are trying to set objectives *before* projects are undertaken. Too often there is a conflict as to whether completed tasks meet acceptable standards. This is precisely what is missing from these statements and the reason that they are unacceptable in their present form. As they stand now there is really no commitment to anything except to undertake a project and get it completed according to a time and cost projection.

Thus, following such a simple formula leads us right into the input or activity trap, which we are trying to avoid with MBO. Apparently the simple approach is too simplistic. The attempt to save work and make it easy to write objectives does not pay off. As usual, you get what you pay for.

CRITERIA APPROACH

Others seek to improve on the simplistic approach by suggesting that the four elements in the formula are too few. If we add a couple more to be sure the statement includes all the information it should, we might have something. For example, one list of "criteria" for a good objective statement says the goal should include:

1. outcome
2. action
3. actor
4. time
5. proficiency
6. measurement[2]

Put another way, this list of criteria is an attempt to be sure that each objective answers three questions:

1. What results do you want to achieve (1, 2, and 3)?
2. How will you gauge the success of your efforts (5, 6)?
3. When will the result be realized (4)?

Here are some sample goal statements using this approach:

- By January 30, to notify at least 60 percent of past due accounts of the amount of debt they accumulated; the percentage to be verified by the accounting department, which will receive from the collections supervisor a list of patients so notified.
- By October 15, the personnel department will develop a systematic performance appraisal procedure of which 80 percent of the concepts will be implemented.

Question: Critically evaluate one of the above objective statements. Determine whether the one you select serves the function of an objective. Does it describe the result desired in a satisfactory manner? Does it indicate the direction and degree of change from the present?

Answer:

Again, no matter which of the objective statements you chose, you should have noted that the statement, as it stands, still does not get at the result that made the task worth doing. As it stands, the statement permits telling whether the task is done acceptably, but why do the task in the first place? What result is the task geared at improving? How do you know whether you should continue the task? For example, what happens if none of those who receive notices about accounts due actually pays? Shall we simply send another notice 60 days later? What is the real result we are after: having notices mailed? What is the notice for? Would we not be further ahead if we made the objective something to do with reducing the basic problem? We must beware of getting lost in the details of the activities of recording and notifying, instead of moving toward solutions.

SATISFACTORY CONDITIONS APPROACH

Others recommend a different approach to fixing the simple formula method of setting objectives. Realizing that the formula often leads to activities or the mere identification of a project to be undertaken, they encourage a two-step approach: (1) state your aim using the formula, and then (2) add this phrase:

> This objective will be considered achieved when the following conditions exist:
> 1. ______________________________
> 2. ______________________________
> 3. ______________________________
> etc.

The idea is that the conditions listed provide a way of telling if the activity was accomplished in a satisfactory manner. Here are two examples written with this approach:

- To work toward improvement of communications between department heads and administration. This objective will be considered achieved when the following conditions exist:
  1. At least four staff meetings have been held on a scheduled basis per quarter.
  2. Informal sessions have been held on an informal basis each quarter.
- To review the committee structure of nursing service and develop a revised approach by January 15. This objective will be considered achieved when the following conditions exist:
  1. Areas or topics needing standing committees have been identified.
  2. Purposes of ad hoc committees have been defined.
  3. Procedural matters pertaining to committees (such as authorization, objectives, reporting schedules, and membership) have been revised.

Question: Critically evaluate one of the above objective statements. Determine whether the one you select serves the function of an objective. Does it describe the result desired? Does it indicate the direction and degree of change from the present?

Answer:

You should have noted that each of the above objective statements still does not adequately describe the goal line because the list of "conditions" sought is simply an itemization of the steps to be done in accomplishing the project. They are themselves subtasks to be performed. For example, scheduled staff meetings are held and informational discussions are available. How does that necessarily demonstrate that communications are any better? Again, these are probably necessary steps connected with improving communications, but is it not possible to have all kinds of meetings and still not communicate?

A REMINDER ABOUT STYLES OF SUPERVISION

At the rate we are going, it seems that in order to correct the oversimplification of the simplistic approach it will be necessary to include in the objective statements all kinds of information about who, what, when, where, and how. But as we seem to be moving in this direction, you should be reminded of our earlier discussion about styles of leadership and our avowed intent to use MBO in a way that builds what Peter Drucker calls "self-control" on the part of those responsible for accomplishing results.

One of the earmarks of autocratic supervision that we discussed was "close supervision," involvement by the superior in all the details of who, when, what, where, and how *when such is not necessary*. To decide that every objective must cover the details of who, what, when, where, and how is liable to foster continued close supervision. Sometimes it is helpful and even necessary for both parties to discuss these details and have them all recorded in the objective statement, but not always.

This suggests that we might need "different strokes for different folks" and different approaches for the same person, depending on the nature of the objective under consideration. Hence we should take the time and trouble and work (and not apologize for it) to learn different ways of stating different kinds of objectives. In this and the next four chapters, then, we will discuss different types of objectives in the belief that one simple approach will not do; a different format is necessary for some, depending on the type of objective involved.

CATEGORIES OF OBJECTIVES

Table 9-1 outlines two major categories of objectives, each of which is further broken down into classes. Note first the two major categories: job related and personal development. When the simplistic, one formula for

Table 9-1 Categories and Classes of Objectives

Class	What It Concerns	Type of Commitment
Category One: Job Related		
Routine (regular)	Normal work output	To meet standards
Problem-solving	Results below par	To find a solution
Innovative	Something new/change	Added benefits
Category Two: Personal Development		
Technical/professional growth	Knowledge, skills, attitudes	Effort to meet a need
Managerial growth	" "	" "
Total human growth	" "	" "

all approach is used, an important motivating factor is lost. This is brought out by the very naming of these two broad categories.

The point can be clarified by asking: to which of the following two requests are you liable to respond more favorably:

1. "Joe/Sue: it's that time of year again when we're supposed to set objectives. Next Tuesday at two o'clock I'd like you to come into the office and bring with you a list of the objectives to which you intend to commit yourself for the coming year. We will go over them together to see what it is you feel you should be doing in living up to your responsibilities. . . ."
2. "Joe/Sue: it's that time of year again when we're supposed to set objectives. Next Tuesday at two o'clock I'd like you to come into the office and bring with you a list of the objectives to which you intend to commit yourself for the forthcoming year. We want to go over them together to see what results you're going to produce on the job and also what you intend to do to contribute to your own personal growth and development."

Let us answer our own question based on reactions observed over and over with client organizations. The first request tends to make you feel challenged to justify your continued existence as a member of the group. It suggests that your superior is playing "top executive" again, checking up on you, or at least interrupting you in your professional pursuits to fill out a form simply because "it's that time of year again." The second request at least recognizes that what you are planning for your own personal growth and development is as important to the superior as the results you are producing on the job. As a matter of fact, the linking of the two (job-related results and personal growth) well might indicate a recognition on the part of the superior that you see a connection between them, that you want to be sure your job contributes to your professional growth, and that, in turn, your personal growth could serve to improve your own performance on the job.

In a word, the very identification of two categories of objectives serves to "turn you on" more to the work of developing objective statements. You see somehow that you are going to get something out of all this, that it is not simply to fill out forms, that it is not only a chance for the "boss" to check up on you. All this is lost in the simplistic approach.

Let those who think that this cannot be—that invitations such as the second one are Machiavellian, that superiors don't have the time or the inclination to really be concerned about their workers' personal development—ponder this question: What organization can grow any faster than its key people?

Definition of Classes of Objectives

Table 9-1 further subdivides each category into different classes. Let us focus on the job-related category. This category will occupy us for the rest of this and for the next three chapters. We shall return to personal development objectives in Chapter 13.

The three classes of job-related objectives come from a suggestion of Peter Drucker that your time on the job is probably devoted to three types of concerns (KRAs).[3] Some of your time is spent on repetitive, routine, regular, reoccurring, bread-and-butter operational concerns. These are the normal work output of you and your group. Objectives covering these responsibilities are called *routine objectives*. If you are a department manager, the day-to-day operational concerns you face deal with such matters as selecting and training personnel, assignment of work, development of improvement plans, and evaluation of the effectiveness of subordinates (in preparing meals, cleaning rooms, transcribing charts, etc.). If you work in the controller's office, your day-to-day, repetitive concerns deal with collecting money, paying bills, retiring debts, generating financial reports, helping prepare budgets, and analyzing reports on expenditures.

Question: Review the list of KRAs developed during the previous chapter. Copy below those that might fall into this class of routine, repetitive concerns. Remember that routine does not mean unimportant, just that it is ongoing. It was part of your job last year, you're responsible for it this year, and you're likely to have to answer for it next year, too. We're looking only for the one- or two-word phrase.

Answer:

You should have listed here those items from the list of KRAs that seem to be ongoing in nature. Most of them will come from your job description. As a rule, the routine items answer questions such as the following:

- Why is my position needed?
- What am I on the payroll to accomplish?
- What results would not be accomplished if my position were eliminated?
- What authority does my position have?
- On what results do I spend a good deal of time?
- For what are my subordinates responsible?
- What results (products, services, advice, controls) constitute the normal work output of me and my group?

Part of your time is also spent solving problems. Here we are not referring to the fire fighting that we are trying to avoid in being results-oriented. When you are results-oriented, problems are not always headaches, obstacles, or interruptions on the job. When you are results-oriented, problems concern outputs with which you are dissatisfied. Problems concern those KRAs in which performance is currently not meeting a satisfactory norm. For example, if you are supposed to have an average volume of 26 x-rays per hour but your average is 20, you have a problem in productivity. If you're supposed to have no more than .5 percent medication error rate and you are at 2 percent, you have a problem with medication distribution. If you are averaging $50.45 per worker more per month overtime than your budgeted amount, you have a problem in overtime control.

Problems, then, refer to areas for which you are responsible but in which current performance is not at an acceptable level.

Question: Review the list of KRAs developed during the previous chapter. Copy below those that might fall into this class of problem areas because present performance is unsatisfactory. You might help yourself by simply completing this sentence: "I am dissatisfied with our present level of ______, ______ and ______."

Answer:

You should have listed here those result areas you are having a difficult time controlling, those in which performance has fallen below your previous norm, below that of comparable departments or units, below standards set by yourself, by professional groups, by accrediting institutions, by local area practice.

At times you will find yourself saying, "I really do not know whether such and such a performance level is acceptable, so how do I know whether it's a problem?" This suggests that we must know acceptable norms for all our areas of responsibility. Otherwise we do not even know what is under control and what is out of control. This is one reason why we customarily recommend setting norms for all routine areas of responsibility first and then moving on to others. It is normal to find we do not know the acceptable norm for some areas the first time we ask these questions.

Finally, part of your time is spent on *developmental, innovative* areas, things you're doing because of their long-term impact on your operation. They deal with change: either some new project you are getting into for the first time, some new way of doing an old project, some unique program understood to be a one-shot deal. You are engaged in them, however, because they add to the results of you and your work group. We call these your innovative objectives. They are the exact opposite of the routine or repetitive.

You are responsible for creating a new training program, for finding an improved way to perform a patient procedure, for the construction of a new building, for automating some procedure, for offering some new service, for rewriting a manual, for reorganizing departmental reporting relationships. Each of these is an innovative area because (it is hoped) it is not what you do over and over again.

Question: Review the list of KRAs developed during the previous chapter. Copy below those that might fall into this class of innovative objectives.

Answer:

You should have listed here all those areas that you tend to think of in terms of: "I'm going to inaugurate, to innovate, to begin, to design, to implement, to rearrange, to rewrite, to study," and so forth. These words are the tip-off that you are in the area of innovation.

Commitment for Each Class of Objectives

Table 9-1 lists a final column for each class of job-related objectives. A different type of commitment is called for between superior and subordinate during the objective-setting negotiation session, depending on which class of objective is under discussion. It is because a different commitment is called for that a different format is needed to capture this commitment in writing.

When you and your administrative superior are negotiating objectives for your routine areas of responsibility, you are trying to describe in a mutually satisfactory manner how you will know the results are what they ought to be. Whenever anything is done over and over, whenever you repeat something day in and day out, year in and year out, whenever you are dealing with some result that is a normal (frequent) output of you and your work group and probably of similar work groups in your own or other hospitals, it would seem that the very repetition after a while provides sufficient historical data to get a feel for what is acceptable. We usually call this a *standard*. Note that it is experience, for which there is evidence, that gives rise to the acceptable standard, not subjective judgment, intuition, or crystal-ball gazing.

The commitment, then, that you and your superior will work out is to a series of standards of performance that will describe the job done in an acceptable manner. You promise to meet (or exceed) such norms. All you really have to discuss is the source of the norm (your own experience or someone else's) and whatever might be going on in your area that might call for a variation from such norms.

Since you're dealing here with repetitive results, since the commitment is simply to meet or exceed previously met standards, there would not seem to be any great need for a lot of conversation or documentation about who, what, where, when, and how. The assumption for routine areas ought to be that you have them pretty well under control and will continue to do so. Nothing is gained by long interrogation about details.

When you come to problem-solving objectives, you will be talking about the two or three most significant areas in which you feel decided improvement is needed to get the situation back under control. It would seem that for these areas it is going to be necessary to do more than reaffirm the level of performance desired. Here, the very fact that you have selected these areas for attention due to present unsatisfactory performance would suggest the need for longer discussion, for examination of the who, what, where, when, and how.

Here the commitment must be to more than definition of standards. Here the logical expectation would be for a commitment to solve the problem, to raise the present unsatisfactory level to one that meets the norms. What must be captured, then, in the meeting of the minds and in the documentation of the negotiation sessions is a detailed analysis of the problem and a detailed plan of action or solution. Success will be measured by solving the problem.

When you get to innovation, you'll be discussing developmental areas that you think will add to results. The innovations are supposed to improve the overall performance of you and your work group. These objectives ought to be stated in a way that emphasizes how the unit will be better off after implementation of your innovations. The commitment will be to those added benefits. Success will be measured by achieving that added payoff.

Question: To ensure that you have the differences among these three job-related objectives clearly in mind, list here the three classes and for each one select a key word that might be used to define or differentiate each. Then for each class select a key word that describes the commitment sought in the objective statement.

Answer:

For routine objectives, you should note the key word is *repetitive* and the commitment is to *standards* of performance. For problem objectives, you should note they are by definition *below standard* and the commitment is to a *solution*. For innovations, the key word is *change* and the commitment is to *added benefits*.

SEQUENCE FOR CONSIDERATION OF OBJECTIVES

So far we have been trying to make the point that different kinds of objectives call for different kinds of commitment and, therefore, different formats for stating them. The three classes are based on the three kinds of job concerns we have. But there is also a deeper consideration behind classification of objectives. It is based on the management theory that as you move from one type to another you climb to a higher level of excellence.

1. The manager who simply takes care of routine areas of responsibility, has the repetitive things under control, has all the square pegs in the square holes and the round pegs in the round holes, runs a tight ship, so to speak—this manager is worth something to the hospital. We value such people.
2. Worth a little more is the manager who is not flustered the minute things go a little out of control; he actually expects this to happen from time to time and is wise in finding ways to get them back under

control and can solve problems as they arise. We usually try to have people around who can do this not only in their own areas of responsibility but who can also help other managers "keep their cool." Some people shape their whole careers around this. We send them from department to department to solve the knotty problems as they come up. They get to be called "troubleshooters." The point is, they are worth more to the hospital.

3. Worth still more is the individual who not only controls routine affairs and solves problems as they arise (both of which deal with the present), but who also looks to the future, who is developmental, innovative, creative. We prize people who are out there in the foreground, helping forge new frontiers, making the breakthrough for which everyone has been searching. The salary administrators say "we put a premium on creativity."

Notice, however, we are not saying that the person who is solely creative is worth more than anyone else. It isn't a matter of "either-or"; it's a matter of "and-also."

Now add to that the question: Where is the fun in managing? In the control of routine, repetitive results? Of course not. The challenge in management is in the areas of problem solving and innovation. But the caution here is that one cannot afford to work with the problems and innovations until the routine areas are first under control.

The real lesson in all this? Start with the routine result areas—define acceptable standards for them first, get them under control—and then you can delegate them to someone else while you turn your attention to the problems and innovations.

This ought to suggest, finally, that even though the threefold classification of job-related objectives applies to everyone, there might be a different proportioning of them for different individuals.

Question: What's the first consideration that might determine how an individual's objectives are divided with respect to being routine, problem-solving, and innovative? And what differences does it make in the proportion of each type?

Answer:

You should have noted from the above discussion that position in the managerial hierarchy is the first consideration. The higher up one is in the management hierarchy, the greater the proportion of the objectives that will be problem-solving and innovative, with a smaller percentage dealing with routine results, whereas the closer one is to first-level supervision (the closer to the trenches where the daily action is), the greater the proportion of objectives that will be in the routine area.

Question: What's the second consideration that should affect the distribution of a person's objectives among the three classes of routine, problem-solving, and innovative? What difference will it make?

Answer:

You should have said that the *function* one has is the second consideration. The type of job one does or the kind of department or work unit one manages will make a difference once we start developing each of these three classes of objectives. By function, we refer to the classic distinction of line versus staff. Line managers are those whose work units produce the major outputs of the organization. In a manufacturing firm, the line departments are manufacturing, marketing, and finance. In a retailing firm, the line departments are the buying and selling areas. In a hospital, the line areas are those providing direct patient care. Staff departments are those present to assist the line in the accomplishment of their mission. They are often thought of as the support departments, the service departments, the auxiliary or ancillary departments.

As you can see from the definitions, the line departments would be expected to have more repetitive, ongoing, routine results, whereas the staff areas, by definition, concentrate on problem solving and being creative as an assist to the line. They do not have a monopoly on this, however. Certainly line departments must be creative and not leave that all up to the staff people. This distinction is offered simply by way of preparing you for the realization you will soon encounter. As you begin to develop objectives you will discover that the difficulty in identifying all three classes of objectives will depend on which type of department you manage.

SUMMARY

This chapter has suggested that the way to develop objectives on paper ought to follow the type of meeting of minds desired between two levels of managers when they sit down to negotiate mutually acceptable objectives. The type of agreement sought seems to flow from the type of result areas under discussion. Some result areas concern job performance directly; others have to do with personal growth or development.

With regard to job-related objectives, three classes seem called for, given the three kinds of results with which most of us are concerned: routine concerns, problems to be solved, and innovative projects. Figure 9-1 serves to differentiate once more among the job-related objectives and to suggest a format for each class of objective, as opposed to the overly simplistic formula recommended by some.

There seems to be a tendency in some organizations for the word objective to refer to something extra. A request to state one's objectives seems to be a suggestion that "We know what your regular job is—that's what you were hired for; now we want to know what your objectives are. How are you going to do more?" In such a way of thinking, there is no room in a list of objectives for routine, job-description kinds of concerns.

Figure 9-1 How to Think About Job-Related Objectives

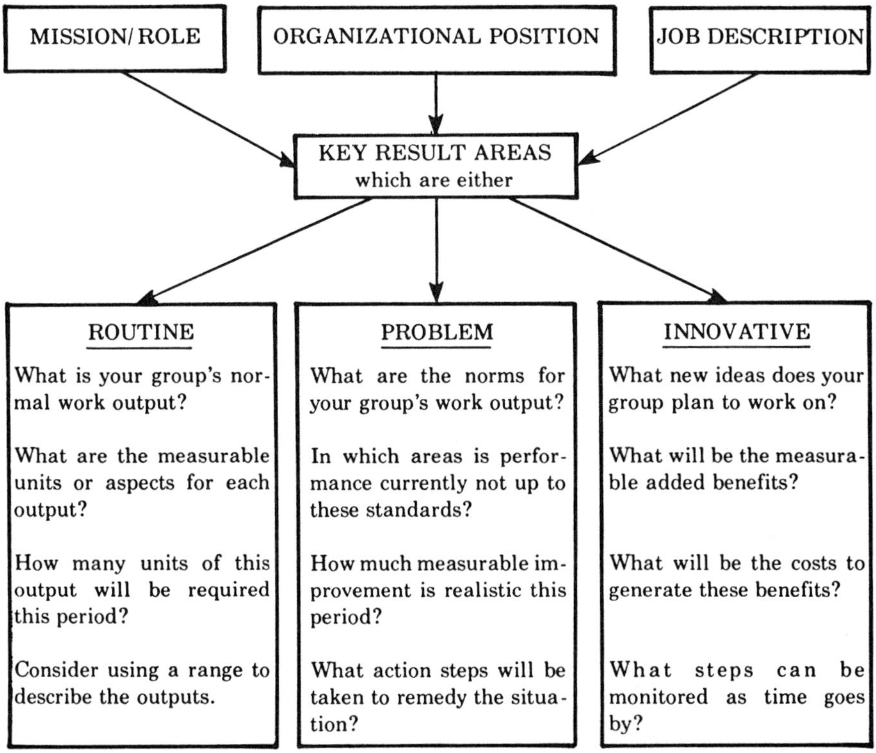

We disagree with this way of thinking. Experience shows that when people get the idea that their objectives concern only the "extras" or the "frills" and then get the idea that their performance review is going to be based in large measure upon accomplishing objectives, the tendency grows for everyone to pay a lot of attention to these extras (because they will have great impact on salary), and no one watches the day-to-day operations. Pretty soon the routine operations cave in. The total list of job-related objectives, therefore, ought to include routine areas as well as problems and innovations.

NOTES

1. George Morrissey, *Management by Objectives & Results* (Reading, MA: Addison-Wesley, 1970).
2. National Laboratory for Higher Education, *MBO Training* (England: David Carpenter Classified Media Ltd, 1971).
3. Peter Drucker, *The Effective Executive* (New York: Harper & Row, 1967).

Chapter 10

How to State Routine Objectives

In Chapter 8 we suggested that there were eight steps to implement this system of management. The first five had to do with developing/stating the objectives in a way that there was agreement between superior and subordinate; the last three had to do with monitoring or measuring progress in achieving the objectives.

In that chapter we also learned how to develop KRAs, the first step in implementation. Chapter 9 was an interruption of the process in the belief that we had to classify result areas before we could go on with the development of objective statements. We are now ready to resume the sequence of steps to state objectives, using a different format for each class of objectives. This chapter will discuss the routine areas; the next two chapters will take up problem areas and innovations.

FORMAT FOR ROUTINE OBJECTIVES

Exhibit 10-1 is the recommended format for stating routine objectives. The columnar approach will emphasize that, in our opinion, the essence of a well-stated objective is not to comply with the rules of composition and syntax. We have been involved in too many objective-setting discussions in which the major disagreements were about grammar rather than substantive ideas. This can be avoided by focusing on the information rather than on the English.

Column 1 is headed Key Result Areas. Remember we are now dealing only with routine, repetitive result areas. In this column should be listed those KRAs for which you are responsible. They fall into this class because of their ongoing nature.

Question: Refer back to Chapter 8 and copy onto the first column of Exhibit 10-1 those KRAs you selected for yourself as being routine.

Exhibit 10-1 Format for Routine Objectives

(1) Key Result Areas	(2) Indicators of Success	(3) Present Level	(4) Desired Level		
			Min Acc (worst)	Exp Ave	Max Prob (best)

INDICATORS OF SUCCESS

Now take each KRA in turn and determine how to measure success. The KRA tells you *what* you are trying to measure; the indicator column (2) on Exhibit 10-1 tells you *how* to measure it. You are deciding here what yardsticks you wish to apply as time goes by to determine that you are getting what you want. "As measured by . . . ?" could be an alternative heading for this column, as this is the next logical question to settle between matched pairs of managers.

Several times it has been urged that every objective must be concrete, must be measurable. We tried to avoid the phrase "must be quantifiable." If there is a difference, there must be ways of measurement other than quantification. We also believe with Harry Levinson that often it is these other ways of measuring that are most meaningful to people in setting their objectives.[1] This seems to be even more the case with professionals, such as health care providers.

Experience of others suggests that there are four broad types of indicators of success to apply to different KRAs. These types are found in the four words: *quantity, quality, time,* and *cost.* Take each of your KRAs and ask yourself: "As measured by . . . quantity? . . . quality? . . . time? . . . cost?" Think of each in turn. Find out all the possible ways of measuring the result in question and then select the one or two (or more) indicators that seem to be most critical for you in monitoring that result area for the next time period. This suggests there might be more than one way of measuring success. There could also be differences of opinion between individuals as to which is more critical. You might also change your mind as time passes by.

Let us see some examples of how this works. As we do, notice that we do not list the word *quantity* or *quality* under the indicator column. We put down what it is we are quantifying, units of what? Or we put down the particular quality we have in mind to measure.

Quantity

The thought process normally begins by asking: Is there some quantitative dimension of the results we are seeking? Is there a normal work unit? Can we talk about number of patients served in this responsibility area? Can we count units of production? Is it something we are processing, so that our work is truly a kind of production line, such as number of purchase orders processed, number of requisitions filled, number of forms printed, number of requests answered, number of meals prepared?

Any time you have (or can acquire without establishing entire new record-keeping systems) raw data, you should use these quantitative figures as a way of measuring progress because they provide the most objective sort of information: facts are always facts.

At times you might wish to count the absolute numbers for something. At other times, a percent is more meaningful, since the absolute number might fluctuate widely or really not matter. What might matter is a good "batting average" no matter what the absolute numbers look like. A word or two of caution about percents, though:

Do not use percents as a way of measuring unless you intend to keep track 100 percent of the time that thing occurs. For example, a comptroller with the responsibility for budget control probably should not use "percent of departments over budget" as an indicator of success. This would necessitate recording all actions on all incidents, and that would be unnecessary. All we are interested in is keeping certain undesirable results to a minimum, so he would probably use "number of departments over budget" as the indicator of success. But it would make sense in dietary to speak of "percent raw food wasted," rather than "number of meals discarded."

It will also be a lot easier to express results as an absolute number rather than a percent increase or decrease because the latter approach requires a double computation. You have to find out what the result was and then determine how much of an increase or decrease over the preceding period. It is easier simply to state the objective as an absolute number. Besides, motivationally, it really does not excite anyone to be aiming at a percent, but give them an idea of what that percent stands for in concrete numbers, and watch their eyes light up. Bell Telephone executives found that encouraging people to achieve "a service index of 97 or 98" didn't change behavior very much, but when they translated that phrase to mean, for an example, that the switchboard operator "answer the phone after only one ring," things began to happen.

Exhibit 10-2 lists some typical quantitative indicators found useful by others.

Quality

Next you ought to ask: Is there some quality we are trying to ensure in the result? What quality is it? Are we interested in accuracy? In completeness? In usefulness? Are there standards already existent somewhere (professional auditing standards, joint commission norms, inspection

Exhibit 10-2 Sample Indicators of Success

Quantity	Number patients served or injured or admitted, etc. Number items processed (orders, forms) Number cases handled (referrals, complaints) Number items produced (meals, clean rooms, x-rays) Percent employees participating in various programs Percent employees absent or late or complaining, etc.
Quality	Error rate (tests, medications, x-rays, meals) Labor hours lost due to injury (severity rate) Percent orders without error (pharmacy, maintenance) Turnover rate of employees Percent work redone (or rejected completely) Percent time out of order (downtime) or unproductive Number citations after inspection (or probations)
Time	Number or percent so many days old (bills, charges) Number or percent answered within so many days Number days to complete (reports, charts, audits) Number working days after the end of the month Time elapsed (turnaround time) Frequency each month/quarter
Cost	Dollar cost per item (x-ray, test, purchase, meal) Percent variance from budget Dollars as a line item in budget (e.g., overtime) Dollars saved over previous period Number labor hours to complete each time

checklist items) so we can talk about a rate of rejection, a rate of compliance?

Note that the quality of the responsibility you are trying to measure might be determined by numbers. This is especially true when we use ratios as an indicator of quality. The treatment therapist ratio is a qualitative indicator of the job you're doing in scheduling/staffing. The number of patient incidents is an indicator of the quality of care.

You ought not get into a long discussion as to whether the indicator of which you have thought is really quantitative or qualitative. These terms (as also *time* and *cost* below) are simply thought starters to help you think of indicators. Once you've found the ones you like, these words have outlived their usefulness.

Exhibit 10-2 lists some typical qualitative indicators found useful by others.

Time

A third dimension to be considered in seeking indicators is the time element. In a sense it is true that all objectives have a time consideration. Recall, however, that here we are still talking about routine, ongoing results. Because they are routine and repetitive, these are not the type of results that are going to have a one-time final completion date assigned to them. By definition, we expect them to have to be achieved repeatedly.

Therefore, time will mean such things as: How often do you expect to accomplish the result in the operating period you have in mind? How long should it take to complete the result each time it's done? How much time should elapse between request for service and completion? What should be the turnaround time for the repetitive result to be achieved? How many working days after completion of the appropriate time period should it take for the result to be forthcoming?

If a quick look down your indicator column shows a heavy preponderance of "date to be completed" indicators, you might ask yourself whether you have in fact listed routine result areas.

Exhibit 10-2 lists some typical time indicators found useful by others.

Cost

A final question to ask about possible indicators of successful accomplishment deals with what you are willing to spend to achieve it: Is there a budgeted amount of money to accomplish the result continuously? Is there a standard cost for providing the result? Can you say how many hours of work you are willing to allocate to this result area? Can you estimate what percent of time (labor hours) the result is worth?

Again you can use dollars or numbers as a way of expressing the cost element, but it is a different dimension than the quantity of the result. And since MBO is based upon the belief that it is results that are our only claim on assets, it is always helpful to think of what assets/resources limit us in producing results.

Exhibit 10-2 lists some typical cost indicators found useful by others.

How Many Indicators?

You ought not to conclude from discussion of the four types of indicators that each result area necessarily should be measured by all four. But you might wish to do that in some cases. Whatever number will be needed to monitor progress the way the matched pair wants to monitor it is the right number. You should go through this thinking process and be ready to negotiate which one, two, or more indicators are most critical to watch during the coming period of operation.

Here are some examples of what you might come up with for given responsibility areas:

- A nursing supervisor might be responsible for quality of care, as measured by audit standards not met, number of medication errors per month, or frequency of patient incidents per month.
- The controller might be responsible for financial reports, as measured by accuracy, dates submitted, or helpfulness.
- The purchasing agent might be responsible for purchase orders, as measured by percent filled when requested, standard cost to prepare, or number converted to blanket orders.
- The personnel manager might be responsible for employee record maintenance, as measured by number of errors per quarter, days to complete after quarter ends, or days to respond to request for information.

Managing by Exception

It might help to realize that the management of routine operations is where we can most advantageously make use of the principle of exception. It was indicated in Chapter 9 that the way to measure routine responsibilities is "by exception." The idea is that you want to get these areas under control and delegate them to others so you can turn your attention to problems and innovations. You should return to routine areas only when they get out of control.

This would suggest, then, that the norms you are setting for these ongoing results ought to be expressed in such a way that you will know when they are out of control, when they do not meet the standards. This means you will often choose as indicators of success what might appear to be "negative" measurements. You will often find mention of error rates, complaints, rejected work, deadlines missed, and so forth. The assumption is that the job is done as it should be more often than not, so it should be easier to keep track of the times when it does not meet the norm.

Further, it will often be impossible to count or keep track of the time when results were as desired/expected: we do not even hear about it unless something goes wrong. For example, safety is recorded when it is missing (accident rate); attendance is listed when it is not there (absentee rate); persistency is measured by its absence (turnover rate); filing is done well unless something cannot be found (misfiled). We talk about wrong deliveries, assuming most are right; we isolate errors assuming most work is correct; we speak of a failure rate, knowing most times people and things work as planned.

This is not encouraging people to think negatively; it's simply an attempt to minimize bookkeeping and a reminder to get involved only when tolerances have been exceeded. It is also a recognition that we often cannot measure the result directly but have to resort to symptoms of its presence or absence. Do physicians measure health directly? No, they measure the symptoms of good or poor health by recording temperature, pulse, blood pressure, and so forth.

Nor are we *planning* so many errors or accidents or the like when we choose such indicators. What we are doing is planning *no more than* so many errors or accidents. We are planning to control them.

Some Most Common Indicators

At the risk of appearing to be getting up on a soap box, we would like to offer one final bit of advice before suggesting that you apply all the above to your own routine result areas.

No matter what type of unit you manage, the name of the game is always *to get more output per unit of input.* We all realize effectiveness is more important than efficiency. But we must face the challenge of not wasting resources right here in considering our ongoing, routine responsibilities.

We therefore suggest that every manager has a responsibility to increase productivity. Whether it is the laboratory supervisor thinking of ways to motivate technicians, the data processing manager pondering new systems and procedures, or the executive housekeeper about to prepare the budget for cleaning supplies—all should be aware of the need of managing their operations such that they require fewer assets (machines, personnel, supplies) per unit of output (tests completed, systems designed, or rooms cleaned).

Notice, then, that productivity is always output divided by input. And input is not always labor hours. Inputs include all the factors of production: land, labor, capital. Getting the job done with fewer expendable supplies by the investment in a machine is one way to improve productivity. It might also mean fewer labor hours (especially if there is a machine involved), but not always. It might simply mean a different work flow pattern to save hours or people.

Here we are not really considering such innovative ways of accomplishing the savings in productivity. But we are calling attention to the responsibility of measuring productivity in your ongoing result areas as the one most common indicator shared by many managers. A few more common indicators would include:

- personnel administration, as measured by turnover rate, absenteeism, overtime costs, or repeat discipline cases
- budget administration, as measured by preparation time, variance from budget, or percent of items not foreseen (supplemental dollars)
- service, as measured by average time to respond to request, percent times had to be redone, number of times recommended to others, amount of "repeat business," or number patients served per unit of cost (dollars, hours)
- training of subordinates, as measured by number able to rotate positions, number estimated promotable, percent rating training helpful, or per person dollar amount or time cost

Question: Now return to Exhibit 10-1 and complete the indicator column as it applies to the routine KRAs you listed. Don't be afraid to list several for each KRA: You usually don't know which will be best until you've thought of a few. This is all subject to negotiation later on anyway.

PRESENT LEVEL

You will recall from the institutional objective-setting exercise in Chapter 6 that the place to begin setting objectives for the future is with an examination of the present. Hence, now that you know how to measure the result you wish to achieve, you next determine or estimate the present condition of affairs, using the indicators chosen as most critical for monitoring progress, to find out if any change is to be required. (Present performance could be fine.)

Column 3 is really a mere matter of recording facts. What is the current performance level? This will sometimes mean the level of performance for the most recently completed operational period comparable with the next one you have in mind: a year, a shift, a month.

Let us repeat here something we found happening regarding the hospital objectives: do not be alarmed if you do not know the facts for something. But do realize that apparently you should, since you have selected this as a critical way of measuring one of your responsibilities. Just get busy and start keeping track of it. Remember also to stop keeping records that you do not see as helpful in measuring performance. In the interim you might wish to "guesstimate" what the present performance level is, if only to see if it might be desirable to make any changes.

On the other hand, you could sometimes find, while searching for the facts you need for this column, that you do have records of something almost as good, but not quite the same. This might prompt you to change your mind about indicators to measure results. The previous existence of records might mean that others found this a meaningful way sometime or other to record results.

About the only time you might have difficulty knowing what information to record here will arise when the indicator is a quality not expressible in numbers. The quality of "accuracy" can be stated as a percent or as a deviation. But the quality "thoroughness" or "usefulness" requires some kind of verbal description. The key is to be sure the verbal description is objectively verifiable and not a subjective judgment.

Let us use an analogy and then return to these troublesome qualities. Suppose we wanted to measure the weather. Meteorologists have many ways of measuring it using numbers: they speak of the temperature, barometric pressure, wind velocity and direction, height of the seas or tide, number of tornadoes or lightning bolts, and even the undesirable respirable contaminant rate. Seeing those numbers expressed on a television chart does describe the weather.

But we could also use verbal descriptions to differentiate one type of weather from another for any listener/reader. One day we speak of the weather as being "clear, sunny, cloudless, mild, and pleasant"; but another day we say it has turned "overcast, rainy, raw, and windy." We see a clear change being described, so it suffices to tell us about the weather, even without all the statistics.

Our earlier definition of an objective as the "degree and direction of change we desire from the present" suggests that if our description of the present can be done with adjectives or behavioral statements in such a way that a change would be readily apparent, that will suffice for our purposes. Remember the description must be verifiable objectively (like the weather) and not a matter of subjective judgment.

Let us go back to our troublesome qualities now. Here is how we might describe Column 3 for the result area of reporting, which many of us have as a KRA:

Key Result Area	*Indicator*	*Present Level*
Reporting	(a) accuracy	Projections ±5%
	(b) thoroughness	No unanswered questions about major headings
	(c) usefulness	Statistics only or Reports only on orders carried out

The above describes an ongoing reporting system (financial reporting, nursing reports, etc.) that (a) has a ±5 percent accuracy level in all projections, or (b) has no unanswered questions called for by the major headings on the report, or (c) has limited usefulness due to containing only statistical information or reports on orders carried out exclusively. Next you would want to ask whether this type of reporting is filling the bill. You would describe the desired level of reporting using similar terminology under Column 4. But for now we hope to have shown it is possible to describe the present condition of something even without use of numbers.

Question: Return to Exhibit 10-1 now and complete Column 3 for your routine result areas, using whatever information you have available or making reasonable approximations until you have a chance to verify your data.

DESIRED RESULTS FOR NEXT PERIOD

If an objective is the direction and amount of change desired from the present, and if you have now stated the present level of performance in each of your KRAs, all that remains is to determine how much change and in what direction you desire for the next period. Column 4 is for this purpose.

You will notice, however, that one desired level will not do: a range of outcomes is recommended. This is a rather recent suggestion coming from earlier experiences in attempting to negotiate objectives. Early experience found that, in the effort to emphasize measurable results, there was a tendency sometimes to put down a number just for the sake of having a number. There was not necessarily any commitment to the number selected. Because of the multitude of variables that might influence final results, it was very difficult to get real commitment to any finite number. And this was only human.

Hence in order to build motivation techniques into the system once again, these many variables and their uncertainty should be taken into consideration. Rather than ask for a commitment to a single finite level of performance, why not ask for a range that goes all the way from the minimum acceptable (worst) level for the next period, no matter what those variables might be, to the maximum results probable (best)?

The thinking goes something like this: Assuming the worst about the future and all the things that might hinder performance in this result area, what is the worst level of performance that would still be considered acceptable for you to be doing "a satisfactory job"? How bad can things get and you still feel you are in control of things? What's rock bottom, such that anything below this and you are in trouble?

Now assume that you can control some of those variables in the future and prevent them from having the negative effect on results just considered. Under those circumstances, what is the maximum level of performance you can conceive as probable? What is the best you can hope for and still not be idealistic?

Finally, somewhere in between these two, what level of performance do you honestly expect to be able to make happen for the coming period? What results would be considered average in the typical situation where sometimes the future is not all rosy or all dark?

The definition of the three levels should be agreed upon by the negotiating parties first. This is very important. We believe the headings should be taken literally: "minimum acceptable" should mean just about that—the worst performance acceptable; anything worse is skating on thin ice. "Maximum probable" should mean the best results we can aim at and still be realistic. "Expected average" should not be a mathematic mean, but what is generally anticipated and what can be used as a starting point for budgeting, scheduling, and the like.

It will help to remember that all three points on the range describe results. Hence the minimum column refers to minimum or worst *results*, and maximum refers to maximum or best *results*. Maximum and minimum do not refer to the size of the numbers or percents or dates recorded. Sometimes the minimum number is the maximum results: it depends on what it is we are measuring. In all cases, performance gets better as you go from minimum to maximum. For positive, good, or desirable things the numbers will increase as you go from minimum to maximum; for negative, bad, or undesirable things, the numbers will decrease as you go from minimum to maximum. A little practice will make this apparent: the numbers will seem to reverse themselves for some indicators.

Alternative Uses of the Range

You might find one or more of the following alternative uses of the range helpful, if only to see the motivational benefits of this concept of commitment.

Some will prefer to start the discussion with the present level. Then the negotiating will begin. The parties will discuss, "What inhibiting factors might influence this desired level of performance, and if they happen, what lower level will we be willing to accept?" This sets the minimum. Then they will discuss, "What factors can we envision as having a helpful influence on the desired level of performance to raise it? If we can provide them, what higher level can we realistically commit ourselves to?" This sets the maximum.

In this alternative, the range is thought of as a kind of plus or minus from an original starting point. But the amount plus or minus comes from consideration of hard information about variables, rather than a subjective guess.

Some will prefer to begin the negotiating from the single level of desired performance thought of separately by each of the two parties. One will probably have in mind a level of performance higher than the other. Whoever had the lower level is asked to explain the circumstances that would warrant the lower level of performance. "If the future brings this situation, we'll expect performance to be in one column. If the future brings this other situation, we'll expect performance to be in another column. But if the future turns out to be yet another eventuality, then we'll expect performance to be in still a third column." Then as the future develops and one set or other of assumptions proves out, the appropriate column is where results are expected.

At least one organization we know uses the three columns in connection with probability theory. Managers set three levels of performance, and for each level the two parties consider the uncertainties of the future and what they plan to do about them. Minimum performance describes what they think they can achieve with 90 percent probability; average performance describes what they think they can achieve with 60 percent probability, and maximum performance describes what they think they can accomplish with 30 percent probability.

Question: Return to Exhibit 10-1 and complete Column 4 to indicate the range of outcomes to which you would be willing to commit yourself for all your routine result areas. Be sure to consider carefully what contingencies you would be able to discuss as causing one or another level of performance.

Exhibits 10-3 to 10-5 give some examples of the way your completed Exhibit 10-1 should now look. The responsibilities are for different units and are intended to be illustrative only.

THE NEW BOSS EXERCISE

To acquire some skill in setting these routine objectives and to get a feel for what it is like to have some of your original thoughts about levels of performance or appropriate indicators of performance challenged by another individual, it is sometimes helpful to practice with a hypothetic superior. To do this, simply follow these steps.

Exhibit 10-3 Medical Records Department: Sample Routine Objectives

Key Result Area	*Indicators*	*Present Level*	*Minimum Acceptable*	*Expected Average*	*Maximum Probable*
Patient charts	Number incomplete	775	800	725	625
	% completed w/i 15 days of discharge	92%	90%	92%	96%
	# loose sheets delivered to Med Records daily	200	75	50	25
Audit of charts	% operative reports dictated with 24 hours	75% (est.)	95%	98%	100%
	% incomplete short form discharge summary	30%	80%	90%	100%
	% incomplete nursing discharge summaries	60%	90%	95%	100%
Microfilms	Years still to be filmed	11	2	1	1
Sign-out system	# records not returned w/i two working days	10/mo	10/mo	5/mo	2/mo
	# unaccounted for/ missing	10/mo	10/mo	5/mo	2/mo
Transcriptions	Time between dictation and transcription:				
	Discharge summaries	10 days	7 days	6 days	5 days
	Surgical reports	36 hours	48 hours	36 hours	24 hours
	Consults and H&P's	24 hours	48 hours	24 hours	12 hours
Statistical reports	Adm., disch., deaths, and activities of major depts.	5th of mo	7th	6th	5th
	Analysis of hospital services comparative report of prof. performance	10th day	12th	11th	10th
	Hosp. planning council	15th of mo	15th	12th	10th
	Monthly service reports not ready for meeting	2/mo	1/mo	0	0

Exhibit 10-4 Utilization Review Section: Sample Routine Objectives

Key Result Area	*Indicators*	*Present Level*	*Minimum Acceptable*	*Expected Average*	*Maximum Probable*
Admission certification	# admitting diagnosis rejected	2/mo	2	1	0
	% pts reviewed in 24 hrs	90%	95	98	100
Continuing length of stay	# untimely continuing LOS certification	2/mo	2	1	0
	# pts not achieving average LOS (from PAS norm based on diagnosis) & unexplained	1–2/mo	1	0	0
Discharge coordination	% pts with discharge plans (excluding 1 night stays)	80%	95	98	100
	% discharge plans documented	60%	80	85	90
	% discharge documentations showing pt/family education	40%	70	80	90
U.R. Committee	# meetings held	8/yr	12	15	18
	% Average attendance at mtgs.	60%	80	90	100
Quality assurance (Review of treatments)	# additional diagnoses for which standards of care are set up	3/yr	4	5	6
	# problems or deficiencies per unit	1–2/mo	2	1	0
	# items overlooked (not reviewed)	1–2/case	1	0	0
	# problems identified and solved with documentation	—	1/yr	2/yr	2/yr
	Frequency of meetings with physician advisors	daily	daily	daily	daily

Pick yourself a partner for the purpose of this exercise. It need not be someone who knows a lot about your work. Sometimes it is even better to work with someone who knows little about your area of work, so as not to bring preconceived ideas into the discussion. You are looking to be challenged.

Explain briefly to this "new boss" a little about the nature of your unit and the work that goes on there. A quick sketch of the organizational alignments ought to suffice. Now take Exhibit 10-1 or a reasonable fac-

Exhibit 10-5 Sample Routine Objectives: Nursing Division

Key Result Area	*Indicators*	*Present Level*	*Desired Level*		
			Minimum	*Average*	*Max*
1. Quality patient care	A. Nursing process				
	1) Assessment completed within 24 hours of admission	65%	75%	80%	85%
	2) Care plans begun within 24 hours	65%	75%	80%	85%
	3) Discharge planning documented on discharge	60%	75%	80%	85%
	B. Primary nursing units	2	4	5	6
	C. Patient classification system implemented	All med/ surg units	Critical care units	C.C. Units—A.R.U.	C.C. Units A.R.U. Special Care
	D. Medication errors/month	40	40	30	20
	E. Harmful incidents to patients/ month	50	40	35	30
	F. Staffing (nursing)				
	1) % ratio professional/ nonprofessional	54/46	60/40	65/35	70/30
	2) % RN/LPN vacancy/ budgeted FTE (70–80% occupancy)	10%	10%	8%	6%
	3) % permanent float pool/ staffed FTE	3%	4%	5%	6%
	4) # outside pool FTE/ month				
	– 70% occupancy	—	5	6	7

Exhibit 10-5 continued

Key Result Area	*Indicators*	*Present Level*	*Desired Level*		
			Minimum	*Average*	*Max*
	70–80% occupancy	18	16	10	8
	+ 80% occupancy	—	18	16	14
	G. Discharge planning				
	1) Develop referral effectiveness measure for Social Work Dept.	—	5/1/80	3/1/80	1/1
	2) Research studies—increase mean for both nurse and patient nurse mean: patient mean	3.8 nurse < patient	4.2 nurse : pt. same	5.0 nurse > pt	5 —
	H. Research projects completed	2	1	2	
	I. New patient education programs	1	2	3	
2. Human resources	A. Turnover rate—Nursing personnel	21.5% (1978)	22%	20%	1
	B. Time to fill vacancies	—	6 wks	4 wks	2 wks
	C. Self-learning packages developed	3	6	8	1
	D. O.R. Orientation program implemented	—	6/1/80	3/1/80	1/1
3. Public relations	Number of articles published	1	1	2	
4. Department development	JCAH requirements for social work met	—	7/1/80	5/1/80	3/1
5. Support services	A. Pounds of linen/ patient day	—	12	11	1

simile and begin reviewing with your new boss what you believe to be some of your KRAs. Your partner's role is to be sure that they are repetitive, that they are significant, and that they are results rather than inputs or activities.

Explain the indicators you selected as most critical in your job for the next period. Be willing to negotiate if your new boss might think that from his/her point of view some other ways of measuring performance might be more significant. Describe the present performance levels. Be sure you are drawing upon facts and not supposition. Discussing it aloud should tell you if your description does not clearly define the present situation.

Negotiate desired levels using the range concept. Be sure you base your estimates on assumptions you can clearly describe. You need not write down a lot of such details, but you would want to discuss them. Your new boss will suggest different assumptions about future variables, which should make you willing to alter your original desired levels. Be flexible, but insist on commitments about contingencies as a condition for making commitments about different levels of performance.

CRITICAL ANALYSIS EXERCISE

It might be helpful in sharpening your skills not only for the correct stating of your own routine objectives, but also for the correct reaction to proposed objectives submitted to you for negotiation by subordinates, if we close this chapter with a few sample objectives for you to analyze critically. Assume you are asked to sit down one-on-one (we never do it by written memo alone) with persons who submit the following objectives.

Question: After each of the following "objectives" write your critical analysis of how well it fulfills the definition of a routine objective. Try to improve on those that can be salvaged. (Our comments follow the complete list.)

Sample 1: To coordinate the management of all training for new employees so they can become efficient in less time.

Answer:

Sample 2: To enlarge participation in the fire drill program.

Answer:

Sample 3: To add copying equipment in the dietary department.
Answer:

Sample 4: To investigate the possibility of making a bid to host the next nursing league convention.
Answer:

Sample 5: To work with the new nursing graduates.
Answer:

Sample 6: To increase support for the United Fund drive as measured by the percent of employees who participate.
Answer:

Sample 7: To develop a program of preventive maintenance of all machinery within three months after installation.
Answer:

Sample 8: To improve the department by fulfilling the duties of department manager as outlined in the administrative bulletin.
Answer:

Sample 9: To improve the effectiveness of the affirmative action program as determined by (1) increased employment of nonwhite males; (2) increased employment of nonwhite females; (3) increased employment of females in management positions; (4) increase in nonwhites who are promoted.
Answer:

Sample 10: To provide more timely information on capital budget status.
Answer:

Sample 11: To maintain posted office hours for purposes of hearing employee grievances.
Answer:

Sample 12: To decrease the employee turnover rate by at least 10 percent.
Answer:

Comments

We would offer the following critical comments and suggestions, which you can compare with your own reactions to the dozen sample "objectives."

Sample 1: This looks like a sentence from a job description; at best it is a responsibility. The words *employee efficiency* might be considered a KRA, which then needs an indicator of success and levels of performance. The coordination part of the sentence is just about a paraphrase of the job title and should remind us not to try to measure the whole job in its entirety.

Sample 2: This statement lacks specific measurement. The fire drill program is the KRA; amount of participation is the indicator; we need a present level and a desired level to tell whether the objective is achieved.

Sample 3: This is strictly an input. Why more copying equipment? How will we know the new equipment does what it's supposed to? Are we trying to provide more service; if so, how much? Are we trying to reduce waiting time for copying service? If so, how much, so we'll know how much new equipment is warranted. Once again, it is results that are the only reason to claim resources.

Sample 4: First, this is hardly a repetitive item: you won't be doing this over and over again. Further, as it is expressed, it is just an activity. What results will be enhanced by the investigation and then by the convention, if it comes off? Why have the convention here? This is a program that is thought to contribute to something, but what? How will we know we are better off? How will we measure success?

Sample 5: This is strictly an activity. It might have come up as a result of someone's realizing he/she should spend more time with the new employees. But why? What result will be enhanced? How will we know the time was spent in a worthwhile manner?

Sample 6: Employee participation is commonly accepted as one valid indicator of the KRA "United Fund drive." We lack a precise commitment as to how much, however. And the thought that the percent of participants is the only way to monitor progress is probably one of those instances in which someone forgot that the ultimate result is contributions.

Sample 7: This is all too common in that it cites only an intention and a time deadline. How will we know if the program was "developed"? Will a one-page report be adequate? A 100-page report? We need some more valid measure that the result was achieved, some test of what difference it makes, and how we will know when it is completed satisfactorily, that it worked.

Sample 8: This is about as meaningless an objective as you'll ever see. It simply says the manager will be a manager. Objectives are supposed to tell us how we know the person is fulfilling his/her responsibilities. This one can't be fixed. It needs to be scrapped and a new approach taken.

Sample 9: This one seems much better because it is more precise. The KRA could be Affirmative Action Program and 1 to 4 set indicators, but they are without definite standards. This objective would be improved by using the columnar form instead of the paragraph form, since the column headings would be a reminder that a commitment is needed:

			Desired Level		
KRA	*Indicators*	*Pr Level*	*Min.*	*Avg.*	*Max.*
Affirmative Action Program	1) % nonwhite males employed	?	?	?	?
	2) % nonwhite females employed	?	?	?	?
	3) % nonwhite female mgrs employed	?	?	?	?
	4) % nonwhite promoted	?	?	?	?

Sample 10: This is another responsibility. There is an admission that records should be kept. The question of measuring the accomplishment of this duty is not faced. How timely is timely: daily, weekly, monthly, quarterly? What difference will it make? What change is desirable? How will the information be used?

Sample 11: Again, a mere responsibility or activity. How extensive hours? More important, how will we know what results hearing grievances are supposed to accomplish? Do we hope to see improved performance because of them or improved behavior of some other kind (reduced complaints)?

Sample 12: Finally, we have an almost complete objective. The KRA is unspoken but must be something to do with "personnel administration"; the indicator is turnover rate. We do not know the present or desired rate except that the next year it is to be 10 percent less than it is at the present. Why not simply state both present and desired levels so there will not have to be a double computation?

SUMMARY

This chapter has suggested a simple format for expressing routine or repetitive objectives. In the belief that most often you will be on top of the who, what, where, when, and how of routine results, we suggested that for these objectives, you should simply mention (1) the KRA, (2) an indicator of success to be used to monitor progress (quantity, quality, cost, or time), (3) a description of the present level, and (4) a commitment to desired levels of performance (using a range). Very often the exception principle will be used.

NOTE

1. Harry Levinson, "Management by Whose Objectives?" *Harvard Business Review*, July–August, 1970, p. 125 ff.

Chapter 11

How to State Problem-Solving Objectives

The second category of job-related objectives defined in Chapter 9 was the problem-solving type. We defined this as a result area that at the present time falls below some accepted norm. There are several points about these "problems" worthy of our attention before we get into the mechanics of making objective statements about them.

First, we are not talking here about everything people sometimes call problems. Certainly it is possible, and even common, in too many instances for managers to be "problem-oriented," that is, to spend an undue amount of time moving from one crisis to another. We decried this in the first chapter, where we suggested that MBO is an attempt to focus on objective results rather than one brush fire after another. That is why it is so important here to adhere to our definition of a problem: we are concerned here only with areas where the facts of the matter describe below par performance.

The second point worth noting here is that it is normal to have these problems. It is an everyday occurrence for operations to rise and fall and sometimes to be at an unsatisfactory level. And it follows that if it is normal, then it is no shame to call attention to them with an eye toward correcting them. As a matter of fact, it would be shameful to pretend that this did not happen, to live each day saying, "Everything's fine—no problems at all, boss."

Hence, managers who manage by objectives are constantly looking for these problem areas; they build into their system of management a red flag system that will call attention to them, an early warning system so problems can be corrected before they get out of hand. In MBO a tip-off comes when we note performance falling below what we had described as minimum acceptable performance, a difference large enough to warrant action.

Now how can we be sure we have a real problem and not just a vague feeling of uneasiness, a simple brush fire? The following nine-step model is offered as a way of doing precisely this. We shall (1) enumerate the steps in the model, (2) describe each step in detail, (3) show a few worked-out examples using the model, and then (4) guide you through the process for a problem of your own choosing. The steps in the model are to

1. Identify the problem areas.
2. Determine the present unsatisfactory level.
3. Define a reasonable desired performance level.
4. Isolate the difference between present and desired.
5. Brainstorm possible causes of the problem.
6. Decide which causes are the most crucial.
7. Identify alternative solutions.
8. Evaluate proposed solutions.
9. Make a commitment to a time and action plan.

STEP I: IDENTIFYING THE PROBLEM AREA

Your problem objectives will always concern result areas over which you have responsibility and for which you are therefore accountable. Knowing this, you should be somewhat ill at ease about those areas in which performance is not up to par. Hence, to identify such problem areas, you might simply complete the following sentence: "I am dissatisfied with the present level of ________________," filling in the blank space with the result area that gives you reason to be concerned. Chances are that those areas causing you dissatisfaction are the ones in which performance has fallen off or is not what it should be.

You might not be sure yet that results are below par. It could begin with a simple feeling of uneasiness. It could be a recent report that brings something to your attention or a question from a superior or the pressures building from a busy schedule or the human tendency to rush around putting out those brush fires. Wherever the feeling of uneasiness comes from, simply complete the sentence with a result area. In the next couple of steps you will find out if it is a real problem or not.

Perhaps you just saw another monthly statistical report that shows operating room procedures on the decrease, and you have the feeling that this happens too often, so you say, "I'm dissatisfied with the present level of operating room procedures." Or perhaps you have just read a report comparing the supply cost for nursing stations in the hospital and note that yours is second in a list of 13 in the area of high costs. You might say to yourself, "I am dissatisfied with the present level of our supply costs." Or you are looking over a list of KRAs, such as you made for yourself in Chapter 8, and one jumps out at you because it seems to be the one where you spend too little time or too much time, and you have that feeling of uneasiness again. You might select that KRA to complete the sentence.

To ensure that the rest of the model will have immediate application to your work, let us pause a moment here and ask you to complete this sentence literally as it might fit your job. Remember, pick something to fill in the blank that is something *you* are responsible for, something that is a *result,* not an activity or an input. Do not say, "I'm dissatisfied with the present level of apathy of our employees." Apathy is not a result, but a symptom or cause of something else. If apathy is worrying you, translate that worry to a result area by asking yourself what is not being achieved due to apathy.

Question: Complete the sentence, now, as it applies to your job:
Answer: I am dissatisfied with the present level of ________________
____

STEP 2: DETERMINING THE PRESENT LEVEL

This step is simply a matter of getting down on paper the facts of the situation. If you are uneasy about something, the first thing to do is to ascertain the total facts about the matter. Objectively state the present level about which you are dissatisfied. You think something is happening too often? How often? Are you dissatisfied about costs? What are the costs?

Do not get bogged down in this step with all the reasons behind the present level of performance. You are not looking yet for excuses, real contributing causes, guesses about extenuating circumstances, or even suggested ways of coping with the situation. Here you are simply trying to define the present level of performance. It is important all the way through this model to take each item in turn and not jump all over the place with information. Just define the present level of the area with which you are dissatisfied.

Question: Thinking of the result area you chose in Step 1, write down now: What is the present level of performance?
Answer:

STEP 3: DEFINING A REASONABLE DESIRED LEVEL

This is a matter of stating objectively the level of performance that would be par, the norm, the acceptable level. By definition we said a problem deals with results that are below par; what, then, is the par level or standard for the result area about which you are dissatisfied?

It could be that you had defined this reasonable level earlier when considering routine result areas. Or you might have to determine what would be reasonable for the coming period of operations as a kind of "gap closer," an improvement from where you now are as a portion of the way to the standard. Where might you look to find a basis for your judgment about a reasonable level of performance?

You might use "industry norms" such as Hospital Accounting Statistics (HAS); that is, the level of performance achieved by others doing your kind of work in the same kind of environment—other hospitals in your local area, other departments in your institution; standards set by JCAH, and so forth. Any time there is a professional standard set by professional groups, regulatory bodies, accrediting agencies, and the like, they can usually be useful as minimum levels of performance.

Or you might look at your own previous historical records. Perhaps the present unsatisfactory level differs from what you had regularly been achieving, and you would feel things were back to satisfactory if you simply returned to the previous performance level. (Obviously, as times change, we do not always want to stay with previous performance levels.)

The point of all this is that there should be some basis, some rationale, for what you select as a reasonable desired level, *based on facts,* your own or someone else's. You should not pick a level out of thin air.

Question: Taking the result area you chose in Step 1: What would be a reasonable desired level of performance, and what makes you think it is realistic? (You might wish to express it as a range.)

Answer:

STEP 4: ISOLATING THE DIFFERENCE

As Figure 11-1 suggests, the difference between the present level of performance and the desired level of performance is the size of your problem. Graphically, a problem is the same as an obstacle. The block in the diagram has intruded itself between the two half-circles. The natural state of affairs for a circle is to be a round ball, but this circle has been cut

Figure 11-1 Defining the Scope of the Problem

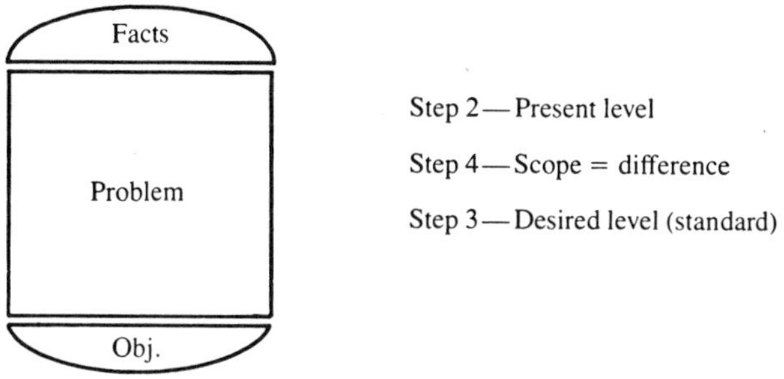

in half by the obstacle called "problem." You want to remove that obstacle. But before you can begin to do that, you first have to define its size. The size of the obstacle will dictate how you will go about removing it.

If you were walking down a path and encountered an obstacle, you would try to determine the size of it before deciding how to remove it. If it were a small stone, you would just kick it out of the way. If it were a large boulder, you could need a crowbar or a bulldozer. If it were half a mountain, you would need some dynamite. Size is what you keep in mind in all subsequent thinking and actions.

So here with problems: you want to define clearly the scope of your problem lest you use inappropriate remedies. You would be surprised how often you start off thinking you have a problem, but after you define the present facts and pick a reasonable desired level, you might find you do not have a problem at all, or perhaps a less serious one than you thought you had.

What difference does that make? Well, the likelihood is that there could be several of these problem areas at any one given time. It then becomes a matter of choosing priorities. One way you prioritize in MBO is by going this far with a series of problem areas; define the scope of several of them and array them one against the others, precisely to determine which one or two are the greatest problems. That is, in which one or two of these areas is the spread between present and desired levels greatest? Those will probably be the areas where the likelihood of making a contribution to the total effort will be greater in the short run, and therefore those might be the areas in which to apply your resources. Since you always have limited time, money, and personnel, you desire to maximize these resources; that means apply them where the return is likely to be greatest. *Your greatest spreads are your greatest opportunities.* How different this is from spending all your time where you simply feel uneasy!

Question: Take time now to determine the difference between the present level and the desired level for the problem you have selected. Is it serious enough to warrant spending scarce resources?

Answer:

STEP 5: BRAINSTORMING POSSIBLE CAUSES

Problem solving is really cause-eliminating. We do not attack problems head-on. We solve them indirectly, that is, by eliminating their causes. The next step then is to identify the causes of your problem so you will have some handles to grab onto in licking the problem.

Because of the emphasis on the participative approach to MBO, we recommend at this stage the use of brainstorming with a small group of associates. The assumption is that you are now dealing with a problem, with some result area in which present performance is below par, in which you have lost control at least temporarily. Left to yourself, results have not been acceptable. Is it not time to seek help then? Is this not the sort of area in which you would expect your administrative superior to be of assistance to you in checking out some of the details? Or perhaps some of the employees who are actually working in the area? Or perhaps some of your peers from other departments whose actions might be contributing to the unsatisfactory situation?

Therefore, why not get together with a small group (five to six persons maximum) and enlist their aid in all that follows? As a matter of fact, they could be a great help in reviewing what you have done so far to be sure you have been objective.

Working with a small group, then, begin to brainstorm what might be contributing causes of the problem. Remember to keep in mind the scope as defined. For example, if 10 percent of the patient charges are sent in late, but you expect there will always be 2 percent of them late as a reasonable desired level, you have only an 8 percent problem in this area. So the brainstorming of causes should be thinking of the extra 8 percent.

You probably do not need to go into all the mechanics of brainstorming, but it might be helpful to remind the group that the principal rule of behavior is "no criticism, negative thinking, or evaluation of ideas yet." This is the idea-*gathering* stage; there will be an idea-*evaluating* stage later. At this point, everyone should simply enter into an exercise of generating the longest list of possible causes. Use a flip chart, a chalkboard, or a tape recorder to keep the ideas up in front of the group.

Let us delay the remainder of this step until we have completely explained the model and looked at an example all worked out.

STEP 6: SELECTING THE MOST CRUCIAL CAUSES

If the brainstorming session is fruitful, you will now have a long list of possible causes for your problem. Among the items on the list will be some right on the mark and some that were helpful to stimulate thought and discussion, but a bit off the mark. We now need to cull the good ideas from the total list. The same small group should then go back over the list and select the most crucial causes of the problem. Peter Drucker calls this the principle of the "crucial few." In any long list of causes there will be a crucial few that account for most of the difficulty.

There is also a fancy name for this idea. It is called "Pareto's Law." Pareto was an Italian economist who noted in his home country that 80 percent of the wealth of the nation was in the hands of 20 percent of the people. (That's true not only in Italy, but also in most nations.) The more you think about it, the more you realize this relationship is true not only in economics, but in most everything. Twenty percent of the people, of the sources, of the staff, of the patients, of the programs, and so forth are responsible for 80 percent of anything that happens, good or bad. It might be called the "80/20 rule."

Eighty percent of your errors come from 20 percent of your workers. Eighty percent of the work done on committees is done by 20 percent of the members. Eighty percent of your turnover comes in 20 percent of the jobs. Generally speaking, 80 percent of the delays in getting anything done come from 20 percent of the people involved.

Of what use is this rule? If you can identify which 20 percent is causing 80 percent of the problem and deal effectively with that 20 percent, you will have solved 80 percent of the problem.

In that group of five or six, you should remember that you are looking for the consensus about crucial causes. This means that in the discussion no one person should be asked to do the ranking. You should avoid the tendency to pose all questions to the person whose problem is being discussed. After all, if that person were aware of all the causes or could properly judge the importance of all contributing factors, chances are the problem would have been taken care of long ago. Do not put every cause to a vote either, as though "majority rule" could always determine which causes are the most crucial.

STEP 7: DEVELOPING ALTERNATIVE SOLUTIONS

When we first defined the different types of objectives and the commitment sought for each during the objective-setting interview, we said that we seek a determination to solve problems. It has taken us this long in the model to get to the solution stage. Why? Because if problem solving is cause-eliminating, we were not ready to think of solutions until now.

Your brainstorming group will want to take the reduced list of crucial causes, post it conspicuously so it will be in full view of everyone, and then attempt to develop alternative solutions by considering each essential cause one by one. The question to pose for the group is "What can be done to eliminate this cause?" A little brainstorming should succeed in developing a few action steps for each cause, all of which should be listed for the group. Do this without discussion or argument about the relative merits of each possible solution.

You are in the idea-*gathering* stage again and should record for later analysis any possible actions that might be taken to eliminate each cause. The next step will *evaluate* the worth of each option. Exhibit 11-1 shows the relationship of these several steps.

Because it's so critical, let's be sure we get the connection.

Question: Where do we get the ideas that will be listed as alternative solutions?
Answer:

You should have said, "From consideration of the crucial causes one by one, because problem solving is cause-eliminating."

STEP 8: EVALUATING THE PROPOSED SOLUTIONS

At this point you now have another long list as a result of the brainstorming. The question becomes, "If we *could* do all those things, which *should* we do?" You certainly would not want to try all the action steps possible, would you?

Question: Why not?
Answer:

You should have said, "Because we want to maximize resources. We have limited time, limited money, limited personnel and probably could not take all those actions even if we wanted to."

But further, we probably would not want to take such a buckshot approach: "Shoot at everything—you might hit something." No, because even if we succeeded in solving the problem, we would not have learned

Exhibit 11-1 Solving the Problem

(Step 5, 6) Causes	(Step 7) Alternative Solutions	(Step 8) Criteria *Cont.*	*Cost*	*Feas.*
* ________	1) ________			
	2) ________			
* ________	3) ________			
	4) ________			
* ________	5) ________			
	6) ________			
* ________	7) ________			
* ________	8) ________			
	9) ________			
* crucial few	ideal	hi	lo	hi

anything. We would be better off with a high-powered rifle shot, even if it takes a couple of efforts. This is what we do in providing patient care; we carefully select a care plan based on judgment, rather than try every medication, operation, or procedure we can think of!

So now you want to work with your discussion group to select from among the alternatives. This time suggest more than a general discussion aimed at a consensus of the group as recommended for cause analysis. Rather, advocate a more rigorous examination of each cause by the application of certain criteria to judge the relative desirability of each option.

The three criteria that have proven most useful in this kind of evaluation are (1) contribution to the objective, (2) cost, and (3) feasibility. Each of these, in turn, has different meanings to different groups and should be well defined before you begin applying them as criteria for selection.

- *Contribution to objective* means how much will this course of action, if adopted, contribute to arriving at the desired level?
- *Cost* can mean out-of-pocket expense, or it can mean net impact on financial position after incremental costs are balanced by improvement in the result area.
- *Feasibility* can mean physical ability to implement the course of action, fit with hospital policy, desirability due to other consequences of an action, legality of the action, its morality, and so forth. The group should define each criterion and keep the same definition in mind while considering all options.

Other criteria are obviously available, depending on the desires of the group or the nature of the problem. For example, in some discussions, time will be of the essence. You might also want to use side effects or impact on morale as a criterion.

Now all that you have to do is select a scale to use. Some people like ranking on a scale of 1 to 10. Others use the simple adjective scale of "high-medium-low" which will be illustrated in the example below. At other times, where you have precise data such as dollar costs, amounts of time, or anticipated quantifiable contributions to objectives, you will want to use that information.

Your group will then fill in the matrix shown under criteria in Exhibit 11-1 with the group judgment. Very often workable alternatives never see the light of day because the people with the problem have decided in advance that they will not work. Their judgment needs to be challenged by others in the group.

When you are through making judgments about each option, you should stand back and find which one or combination of alternatives scored best and, therefore, is your choice. The ideal score should be shown (see Exhibit 11-1) to make selection easy at this time. You then know what course of action to take.

STEP 9: TIME AND ACTION PLAN

Now that you know what course of action seems most likely to help you in achieving your objective (in solving your problem), you are ready to make a commitment in your objective-setting negotiation.

Your time and action plan is simply a commitment to carry out the alternative(s) with the ideal score in the previous step. At this point you are ready to add target dates to (1) initiate the action, (2) complete the action, and (3) evaluate the effectiveness of the action. This is your total commitment and what the entire problem analysis has been designed to accomplish. Sometimes it will take a series of actions. If so, your time and action plan will include a schedule for phasing in each of them and for assessing whether they succeed in solving the problem as intended. If not, of course, it will be back to the drawing board. . . .

SAMPLE USING THIS NINE-STEP MODEL

This model is a lot to swallow all at once. The first time through it is not the easiest sequence in the world to follow, so it might be helpful at this point to put a little flesh and blood on the bare bones by illustrating its use with a problem worked out in this fashion by a group of hospital managers.[1]

The example that follows is such an illustration. We need not be concerned at this time with all the reasons behind all the judgments made (desired level, crucial causes, evaluation of options, etc.). Our purpose is to review the steps in the model, not to second-guess those who worked on the problem. The sequence of steps will also serve as a model to follow for the group assignment that closes this chapter.

1. Statement of problem:
   I am dissatisfied with the current level of linen usage per patient day.
2. Present level:
   21 lbs per patient day.
3. Reasonable desired level:
   13 to 15 lbs per patient day.
   Basis in fact: HAS statistics and local area practice
4. Scope of the problem:
   An extra 6 to 8 lbs per patient day, which can be converted to a considerable dollar expense.
5. Possible causes for the extra lbs.:
   - calibration of scales
   - no written policy about linen usage*
   - lack of awareness of the problem
   - poor laundry management*
   - use of draw sheets
   - theft
   - usage of daily cleaned lab coats*
   - excessive usage of laundered items*
   - weighing procedures
   - changing sheets too often
   - rejected "clean" linen*
   - high labor costs
   - turnover of personnel
6. Crucial few causes:
   the ones with asterisks above
7. and 8. Alternative solutions

		Criteria	
	Cont	*Cost*	*Feas*
a. More disposable in selected areas	hi	?	hi
b. Discontinue draw sheets	hi	lo	hi
c. Lab techs wash own coats	lo	lo	lo

d. Review, rewrite, enforce policies	?	lo	hi
e. Establish criteria to measure manager's effectiveness	hi	lo	hi
f. Better inspection of "clean" linen when packed	lo	lo	hi
g. Mark each unit's and see where excess is coming from	med	hi	hi
h. Discuss at dept head meeting	lo	lo	hi
Ideal	hi	lo	hi

9. Time and action plan:
   a. Immediately review, rewrite (if necessary), and enforce policies.
   b. Study cost of use of selected disposables—2 months.
   c. Discontinue draw sheets (except in ortho wards)—1 month.
   d. Include standard of effectiveness in manager's evaluation starting immediately.
   e. Evaluate effectiveness of these steps in 3 months.

PROBLEM-SOLVING ASSIGNMENT

Now that we have seen the entire model applied to a real problem, you ought to be ready to apply it to one of your own KRAs. You may want to stay with the problem area you first identified at the beginning of this chapter, or you may think of another one. The following sequence of instructions should be followed to permit you to do this with the help of the small group technique discussed throughout the model.

1. Divide into small groups of five or six persons. Deliberately mix with people who are not involved in your own daily operational sphere to get outside insights into your discussion.
2. Working individually, develop a statement of the major managerial problem facing you at the present time. Complete the sentence "I am dissatisfied with the present level of __________________" as discussed above.
3. Select a chairperson who can keep the discussion on the track. He/she should not be hesitant to tell a discussant, "We're not ready to talk about solutions yet; we're still on causes," or "You're criticizing and we're supposed to be brainstorming," and so forth. A time limit for the exercise should also be set so that the chairperson can keep things moving realistically. Ninety minutes from this point on is normally sufficient.
4. Each person should take two or three minutes to explain his/her problem to the small group. The group will ask questions just to

clarify the nature of the problem. The chairperson should not allow anyone to get on a soap box and spend a half hour telling a captive audience about a pet peeve.

5. That group chairperson should then lead in the selection of the one problem that would seem to have the most merit for discussion by the others. Avoid picking a problem shared by many, as though solving it for one would solve it for all. Whichever problem you pick should be seen through the eyes of that one person whose problem it is. Hypothesizing or treating several persons' problems at one time will not lead to concrete judgments.
6. Obtain the use of a chalkboard or a flip chart so the remaining discussion can all be recorded in front of the group and thus allow for objective discussion of information. State briefly the problem by writing down "I am dissatisfied with . . ."
7. Discuss and define briefly the present level.
8. Discuss and define briefly the reasonable desired level. Explain the basis in fact for this as reasonable.
9. Isolate the difference, and be sure the spread is worth the effort it will take to analyze and correct the problem.
10. List the possible contributing causes.
11. Select the most crucial causes.
12. Develop alternative solutions.
13. Choose criteria to evaluate the proposed action steps.
14. Make judgments about each option, using the criteria chosen.
15. Decide on a time and action plan for the best options.

SUMMARY

Problem-solving objectives require more than a commitment to the desired results. Since present performance is below an acceptable level in these areas, the negotiation session should include discussion of proposed action plans to solve the problem.

This chapter has recommended a nine-step model for determining a plausible solution in problem areas. Emphasis is on participative analysis of the situation, with inputs from a variety of sources to shed light on causes of the present problem and possible actions to improve results.

NOTE

1. For further discussion of the model shown here, cf George Odiorne, *Management Decisions by Objectives* (New York: Prentice-Hall, 1969). For a more exhaustive discussion of a detailed model, Charles H. Kepner and Benjamin B. Tregoe, *The Rational Manager* (New York: McGraw Hill, 1965).

Chapter 12

How to State Innovative Objectives

The third type of job-related objective is the innovative objective. Here again the negotiating interview, which works out each individual's "personal contract," ought to generate a particular kind of commitment or meeting of the minds when dealing with innovations.

You will probably find this is the easiest type of objective to think of because a general tendency for most neophytes is to consider "new ideas" first when asked for a list of objectives. The purpose of this chapter will be to define what we mean by innovation, suggest the real commitment that ought to be captured in the objective statement, and provide an opportunity to practice writing one.

WHAT IS AN INNOVATIVE OBJECTIVE?

To help differentiate this type from the others, let's begin by reviewing our definition of the other two job-related objectives.

Question: What is the distinguishing feature of routine objectives? What are you trying to describe in a routine objective statement?

Answer:

You should have recalled that the distinguishing features of a routine objective is that it is *repetitive;* it concerns *ongoing* result areas in which the output is achieved over and over again. The commitment contained in the routine objective statement is simply a description of the *standards* or levels of performance considered par for the course.

Question: What is the distinguishing feature of problem-solving objectives? What are you trying to describe in a problem-oriented objective statement?

Answer:

You should have said problem-oriented objectives deal with those result areas *where present performance levels fall below the accepted norm*. The commitment you seek in this objective statement is to a *solution*.

Innovative objectives deal with yet a third type of result. They deal with *changes*, with *new things*, with different outputs, either because they are being sought for the first time or because they are unique, special, one-shot affairs. You will know you are in the innovative area whenever your initial thoughts about the objective make use of words such as "develop, initiate, inaugurate, implement, begin, design, create, study, rewrite, reorganize, rearrange, re-almost anything."

Innovative objectives are, therefore, the exact opposite of routine because they are not expected to be repetitive. They were not your measure of satisfactory performance in the past, at least not in the same manner. They are sometimes suggested by problem situations, since they make a contribution to remedying unsatisfactory performance, but they are distinct in that they should describe *new results*.

When negotiating these objectives, you will seek a commitment not only to develop, to begin, to study, and so forth but also to accomplish something as a result of what you develop, begin, study. In other words, you seek not change for the sake of change, but change to bring about some payoff, some benefits, some indication the unit is better off after implementation of the innovation.

Question: What is the distinguishing feature of innovative objectives? What commitment do you wish to describe in the innovative objective statement?

Answer:

You should have said that innovative objectives deal with changes, but the commitment you seek is to produce specific improvements/benefits as a result of that change.

FORMAT FOR INNOVATIVE OBJECTIVES

The recommended worksheet format for innovative objectives is shown in Exhibit 12-1. There are four items of information that need to be covered in the innovative objective. They are indicated by the four subheadings: Idea, Results, Method, and Timetable. As with the problem model, this is to ensure that all the information that should enter into a discussion gets discussed, as opposed to the routine-objective format in which a minimum of conversation would seem to be called for.

Opposite the word *idea* record what the innovative project is. This is normally the way you begin to think about it. You might try answering this question: "What new idea do I plan to install, to suggest, to develop, to study in my area of authority during the next operational period? What new project do I have in mind that goes beyond the repetitive operations of my work unit?" For example, you might answer: "We are thinking of converting to primary care nursing."

Notice this is not the objective. This is only the idea you have. This is the brainchild to which you gave birth when thinking about your responsibilities. This is the name of the project you have in mind. This is the creative thought that crossed your mind as you were driving to work or that you thought of while getting dressed or that woke you up as if a light were switched on in the middle of the night.

The actual objective, the output, is the improvement that gave birth to the innovative idea. This is what you want to record opposite the words *results*. What is the payoff you expect? What are the concrete

---

Exhibit 12-1 Innovative Objective Worksheet

Idea: ______________________________

Results: ______________________________

Method	*Timetable*

improvements/new benefits you think warrant the expenditure of time, money, and energy involved in the new idea? We are going way back to the first chapter, in which we suggested that MBO is a way of thinking about the job that says outputs are the only justification for spending the organization's resources; outputs are the only way to determine whether programs (routine or innovative ideas) are successful and hence deserve to be continued.

Your innovative idea is probably a program you think worthwhile. If you are results-oriented, you'll be willing to say, "I *think* it is worthwhile, but we'll *know* only if it produces what I think it will. Therefore, I'm willing to have the innovation measured by the results it generates. If we achieve thus and so, we're successful; if we don't, the idea sounded good, but just didn't live up to expectations and should be abandoned (or fixed up)."

Thus it is possible to introduce the innovation, to succeed in making the change you have in mind, but to fail in producing the results expected, and therefore fail in achieving the objective. Let us take a common example of innovation these days, the automation of some procedure. Suppose, for example, in the business office there is an innovative objective "to automate the preparing and mailing of patient bills by November 1." On November 2 someone asks the controller, "Did you accomplish that objective?"

His answer is, "Oh, yes. Didn't you notice? Since October 22, all invoices have been prepared by computer and mailed out with computer help instead of by hand." The controller obviously thinks he is a success as far as this objective is concerned.

But you're the fiscal vice-president, and you have been wondering about all this because for the past week you've been noticing: (1) it takes twice as long after discharge to get copies of the bill out, (2) there are three times as many mistakes in posting and mailing as there used to be, and (3) there are four times as many employees and labor hours spent in the process as there used to be.

Question: Is the controller really a success? What was wrong with this objective statement?

Answer:

You should have said that getting it all done by computer was the *idea*, not the objective. The real objective, the intended benefits, should have centered around saving time, reducing errors, cutting labor costs for this procedure. The controller made a change but didn't make any improvements, at least not yet. The benefits should have been stated as the objective.

To achieve any benefits, there are always certain associated costs. The remaining two items on our worksheet are to itemize the costs of the desired benefits. In other words, every innovative objective statement is a miniature cost-benefit comparison. You might think the benefits are worthwhile but only worth a limited investment of the unit's resources. So again you have to ask, "How much are we willing to spend on these benefits?" You might not be better off achieving the results if the costs are too high.

Costs are here itemized under the words *method* and *timetable* because by costs we mean more than dollars. We mean all resources that might be spent: dollar costs, time costs, energy costs, people costs, frustration costs, opportunity costs—any and all costs to achieve the intended results. And those are only the start-up costs. After that, what about maintenance costs, policing costs, abandonment costs (if necessary) later on?

A law of economics and social behavior is that nothing is worth more than you are willing to pay for it. Here, then, we want to be sure that the negotiation session includes a consideration of what the nice-sounding, innovative idea is going to cost. Maybe you just cannot afford it, nice as it might sound. Then, in terms of measuring the success of innovation, the total commitment becomes accomplishing the benefits at no more than the resource costs (dollars, time, energy, etc.) you are willing to allocate to them.

Under *method* should be listed all the necessary steps to implement and track the innovation. This should include actions and expenditures in a step-by-step fashion. Beside each item in this schedule of events should be an estimate of dollar expenditures and a time period or completion date under the word *timetable*. This is to suggest that a simple completion date for the entire project is not enough if objectives are supposed to provide a way to monitor progress throughout the period and not just be targets at which to aim.

Some common items that might be considered for inclusion under the word *method* are listed below. Each item would be supported by cost information (people, dollars, hours, dates).

- research: of the literature,
of other organizations
- formal cost-benefit study (if the project is large enough)

- checking base with others affected
- detailed plan of action
- needed final approvals: administrative,
legal,
financial,
moral
- pilot project or trial run
- evaluation of the test
- implementation
- policing/maintaining
- final evaluation of results

ABANDONMENT

One of the important themes of the management theory underlying MBO is acknowledged in knowing when to *abandon* projects. Many times what seems to be a good idea fails, and perhaps without discrediting the innovator. But to continue to work with that project out of false pride or for lack of a substitute program or because of an inability to measure success (absence of predetermined criteria as recommended here) would be to the discredit of the manager. We must know when things outlive their usefulness or when they never do live up to their promise; then we must abandon them. It is often relatively easy to get something new started up, but it then takes an act of Congress to stop it once it gets rolling.

An example from a familiar field might serve to illustrate. During the first days of the late 1970s' energy crisis, several airlines and airfields introduced an innovative procedure regarding commercial airline takeoffs. Instead of allowing departing flights to back away from the ramp and get in line awaiting takeoff near the active runway, together with 5, 10, 20 or more aircraft, the new arrangement called for a loaded plane to wait at the gate until only two or three planes were ahead waiting clearance to take off. Then the pilot would receive the okay from traffic control to start engines and taxi out.

What was the objective? To make planes wait at the gate? Of course not. That was the innovative procedure or idea. The objective was the expected result: a certain estimated savings in fuel. And once the procedure was implemented, planes taking off did succeed in achieving those fuel savings.

However, after a short time under the new procedure it developed that the costs of the fuel conservation by planes taking off was outweighed by offsetting costs. There were, for example, the losses in fuel sustained by landing planes, which now had no gate to enter, thereby causing a congestion backed up to the active runways. That meant more planes circling overhead at the larger airports (which is the only place where the original problem existed). Then there were complaints and frustration costs of arriving passengers about missing connections, impatience to deplane after a hectic flight, lost bags, and so forth.

Lesson: you can institute an idea but fail because you did not achieve the expected results. Or you can even achieve the results but fail because you exceed what you are willing to spend. In either case you should abandon the innovation, which is exactly what the airlines did.

FINAL EXAMPLES OF THE BASIC DISTINCTION

Before suggesting that you practice writing an innovative objective statement, we might dwell on a few examples of the basic distinction we have been trying to suggest throughout this discussion; the successful implementation of an idea or completion of a project versus the real achievement of the desired results.

Example 1: Some innovations come from consideration of problems and are thought of as solutions to those problems. Suppose you have been concerned about increasing medication errors. After much discussion you decide it might be a good idea to try the unit dose method of preparing medications. Is your objective to package medications? No. That is just the idea; your objective is to reduce errors. You can succeed in the new packaging, but you are not successful unless it produces the desired results of fewer errors.

Example 2: A popular innovation some years ago was the employee suggestion system. If your hospital introduced this program (sometimes today called "quality circles"), was the objective simply to "introduce an employee suggestion plan"? No; that was the innovative *idea*. The objective had to be some benefit to patient care and efficiency or quality of work. It was hoped that if you introduced this type of plan you had some criteria in mind for judging whether it was successful. Most often this was supposed to have something to do with increasing employee participation in bringing about improvements on the job. So, you again hoped to determine some level of increase in quality of care (and how to measure it) or at least some amount of increased efficiency in certain areas or reduction in costs, as a way of showing that the new system was doing what you thought it would.

Exhibit 12-2 Sample Innovative Objective: Medical Records Department

Background Facts:
H & P's are getting increasingly difficult to transcribe:

- doctors are not speaking distinctly
- they are not indicating case numbers, room numbers, etc.
- various subheadings of the report (chief complaint, past history, etc.) are not stated, but left for transcriber to assume or figure out
- last names of doctors (especially foreign-born interns) are difficult to understand (should be spelled out), etc.

Idea: To change our procedure so that, when in doubt, transcriptionist will not guess what to type, but will place dictation in doctor's folder, asking for clarification.

Results: 1) To reduce two-week backlog of untranscribed and half-complete (because unintelligible) dictations to no more than 2 days
2) To reduce to zero the number of corrections of H & P's at time of completing chart.

Method:	*Timetable:*
a) Meet with director of medical education (responsible for interns and residents doing most of this).	15 days
b) Check success of this procedure with other hospital in town.	same 15 days
c) Explain change to transcriptionists with list of items serious enough.	next staff meeting
d) DME to announce change to doctors.	their next meeting
e) Arrange with salesman to give the doctors a demonstration of dictation equipment to train on techniques.	next week
f) In case of unintelligible words, etc. file to be placed in doctor's folder.	starting in 30 days
g) Report to be given to DME each week of all files not corrected w/i 48 hrs.	ditto
h) Monitor progress for 30 days.	60 days from now
i) If successful, repeat annually.	next class of interns

Of course, you also thought about costs, or other results, of the suggestion system if you were complete in your planning for the innovation. For example, you should have been ready to measure the impact on employee motivation in terms of participation (or lack of it). And perhaps you should have included a measurement of type of participation by job category, labor grade, sex, seniority, and the like. What about a measurement of the effect of size of award? How does the amount of cash paid affect participation and quality of suggestions submitted? To judge the success of innovation, should not all these be considered?

Exhibit 12-3 Sample Innovative Objective: Utilization Review Section

Background Facts:
Over the years a variety of methods have sprung up to assess the quality of the services provided by this hospital. We have a quality evaluation program in each department, medical audits done basically by the physicians, nursing audits done by nursing personnel, utilization review done by a cross-section of professionals, and now quality assurance as a new directive for peer review. The aims of these overlap.

Idea: To meld our utilization review program into a hospitalwide quality assurance program.

Results: 1) To reduce the number of quality assessment programs to one.
2) To increase average attendance at UR committee meetings from 60% to 90%.
3) To reduce average LOS to 6.0–6.5 days.
4) To maintain our delegated status.

Method	*Timetable*
a) Coordinators & chairpersons of all assessment programs to meet and review missions and job descriptions	15 days from start
b) Visit 2 hospitals in metro area	30 days
c) Written policy and procedure submitted to med staff & administration	60 days
d) Chief of staff to check with PSRO	75 days
e) Med staff & admin. approval	90 days
f) New dept. created and introduced to all	120 days
g) UR committee mtgs. under new format	120 days
h) Quarterly reports begin, to see that UR objectives still being met	180 days
i) Year-end review	360 days

Example 3: The literature is currently full of admonitions, criticisms, and exhortations about nursing care plans. Professional nurses should make a planned contribution to patient care beyond carrying out physician orders, we are told. Pondering all this, nursing departments are attempting to respond by devising appropriate procedures to provide nursing care plans for patients. But this is just an idea. To make it an objective requires itemizing specific benefits having to do with quality of care, such as reduced length of stay, more patients discharged with certain outcome criteria, more patient/physician satisfaction, and so forth.

Exhibits 12-2 and 12-3 are examples of objectives in the innovative area completed using the format illustrated in Exhibit 12-1.

Now it's time for you to practice. Exhibit 12-4 is intended as a worksheet so you can not only see the basic distinction we have been discuss-

Exhibit 12-4 Innovative-Objective Worksheet

Idea: ______________________________

Results: ______________________________

Method	*Timetable*

ing but outline the major steps of an innovative objective, including a method and a timetable.

Question: Answer the following question using the worksheet in Exhibit 12-4: What new idea are you planning to install, to suggest, to study in your area of authority during the coming operational year? Let your thoughts be challenged by someone so they are specific. Avoid "results" stated without a commitment as to specific measurable amounts.

SUMMARY

This chapter has dealt with innovative objectives, defined as those for which you intend to do something completely new or somehow effect a change in the operation. By considering innovative objectives as deserving of a cost-benefit analysis, you will obtain agreement ahead of time on measurable benefits of the change to indicate true progress has really been made, as well as the time, money, and effort the organization can afford to achieve those benefits.

Chapter 13

How to State Personal Development Objectives

In an earlier chapter we suggested that one of the ways to motivate subordinates to set themselves challenging objectives and do the work it takes to prepare to negotiate these objectives is to emphasize that this system is going to help not only the organization to grow and develop, but it is also going to help the people in the organization to do the same. Practically speaking, however, the time to discuss personal development is not at the same time you negotiate work-related objectives, but on the occasion of the annual performance review. For this reason we are deliberately locating this chapter near the chapter dedicated to a discussion of results-oriented performance appraisal.

Since no organization grows any faster than its key people, managers are also interested in discussing personal growth with their staff. With both parties interested in the topic, it ought to be easy to discuss and encourage personal development.

Yet it often happens that introduction of this topic is greeted with animosity or defensiveness. Some people seem to think that personal growth is a subject you get into only with poor performers. We would like to posit the thesis that everyone needs to grow, that personal development is a normal process, that personal development objectives are a means of fostering that growth, and therefore that discussion of personal development objectives is a privilege to be looked forward to by everyone.

Figure 13-1 is an attempt to prove the universal need for personal growth by pointing out three types of development needs. As a manager it is your responsibility to periodically ask the questions in Figure 13-1 about each of your subordinates and make the judgments that they call for. In doing so, you will find that each of your staff, at a given moment in time, is either an unsatisfactory performer, a career person not interested in or qualified for promotion, or an upward mobile (types I, II, or III in the diagram).

Figure 13-1 Three Types of Development Needs

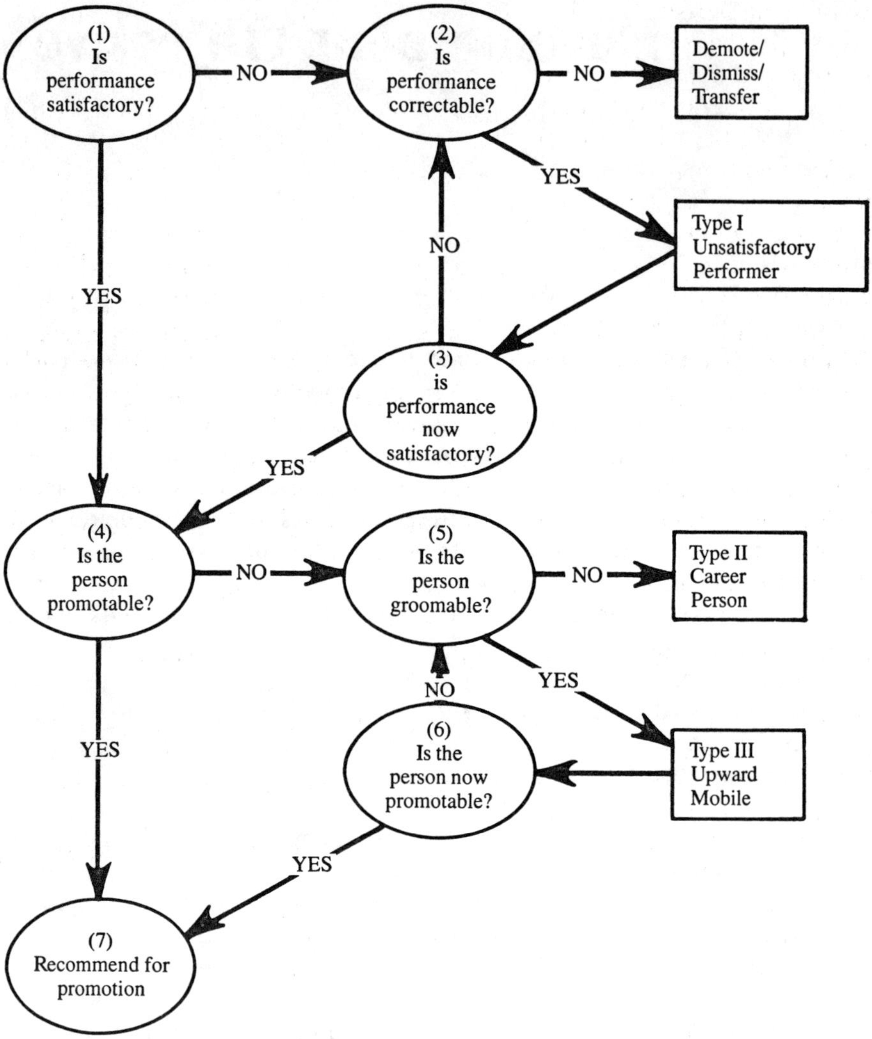

Source: Reprinted from *Coaching* by Arthur X. Deegan, II with permission of Addison-Wesley Publishing Co., 1979. See that text for detailed explanation.

This is not to suggest that individuals are getting labels placed on them that cannot be removed. People do move from one type to another depending on personal motivation, effort, need, or interest. But at any moment a person is at one stage or other of development and consequently in need of one type or other of personal development objective.

Unsatisfactory performers are in need of development objectives that will enable them to raise the present unsatisfactory performance to an acceptable level. Discussion will help identify areas of weakness so that improvement can be made.

Career persons, those who have found a niche for themselves, who aren't really going to get ready for additional responsibilities but are doing a satisfactory job at present, still need to grow if only to keep abreast of developments in the job. No job stays still. No professional can afford to become obsolete. Continuing education is an ongoing effort to prevent a person from losing touch with new developments of technology, of procedure, of systems, and the like. Discussion here will help identify ways to grow at least to keep up with new demands of the job.

The upward mobile, who wishes to be prepared for promotion opportunities, is in need of development objectives precisely in order to grow into the next level position. Discussion will explore ways to get ready for these new responsibilities before they become a reality.

FORMAT FOR PERSONAL DEVELOPMENT OBJECTIVES

Just as the job was deemed too all encompassing to allow a single method of measurement and we therefore broke the job down into its component parts called key result areas that could individually be measured, so personal development is too amorphous to be measured *in toto*. Personal growth probably takes place in one or more of the following three areas:

1. growth in a technical or professional career
2. growth in a managerial career
3. growth as a total person

First is growth in one's technical or professional career. Today is the age of specialization. Your people are not only health care specialists, they are probably trained in detail in one or more of the professions, subprofessions, or paraprofessions that abound in our hospitals today. Each one is in nursing, medical records, radiology, accounting, food services, engineering, and so forth.

And each of them probably has the feeling most of us have from time to time that there is so much going on in our field of specialization that if we don't make a concerted effort to keep our heads above water we will drown in a sea of developments taking place in our chosen fields. The only way to keep up with such developments is to make a commitment to oneself to do so and to measure as time goes by what growth is taking place.

Second is growth in one's managerial career. There is argument about whether management is an art or a science: it is probably both. As such it is undoubtedly changing, growing as much as any of the other specialty fields we have mentioned. And again managers often get the sensation that there are so many meetings on management they would like to attend, so many books and journals on management they would like to read, yet there are not enough hours in a day to get to them all.

It would be as silly to say about management, "I have a degree in management" or "I took a course in supervision" as an excuse not to grow as a manager as it is to say about nursing or accounting, "I have a degree in that, so I don't have to study it any more."

One needs to make a commitment to oneself to grow as a manager just as one does about a specialty field and set objectives to measure that growth.

Third is total human growth. This is a final area that itself could be broken down into many subsections. It is a reminder that we are humans and not professional machines. It is an attempt to avoid being a "workaholic," the kind of professional or manager who eats, drinks, sleeps the job, the job, the job, but who cannot relate to other humans for lack of growing as a person first. Recently there is a new acronym for this kind of person. We call him/her an ACORN. That stands for an addictive, compulsive, obsessive, really nutty person.

To prevent becoming an ACORN, we want to make every effort to grow as a total human by paying attention to other dimensions of our humanity besides our work life. We think of hobbies, sports, culture, ethics, news, civic events, history, and the like. We want to become an OAK, which means an open, adaptive, knowing person.

The discussion will sometimes turn to mention of a developmental need for an individual that touches on health, hygiene, or hobbies. Maybe the biggest favor you can do some people by way of personal development is to convince them to relax, take a vacation, learn to smile, develop interests outside of the job. We have seen executives sincerely commit themselves to an objective "to golf twice a month," or an objective "to take up rock collecting" or "to learn to swim." Obviously they made sense only because there had been an earlier identification of a need for distraction or a need for exercise or just plain a need to devote their energies to something divorced from the job so they can return to the job fresh and ready to work and not "burned out" from thinking of the job all weekend long.

A word of caution about such objectives, however, because of what some people might do with this type of information. In one of the states of the United States there was an executive decision some years ago to implement MBO in all state departments. That meant that all state executives received training in MBO as explained in this book. That was followed by all executives committing themselves to all the classes of objectives we have been talking about, including personal development.

Part of the system was a reward program under which bonuses were paid for successful accomplishment of objectives. So at the end of the first year on the system, performance reviews were held, and bonuses awarded to those who were most successful in achieving their agreed-upon objectives. A major daily newspaper in the state published headlines to the effect that executives were being paid bonuses for golfing twice a month!

Indicators of Success

When we practiced writing job-related objectives, we followed the identification of KRAs with selection of critical indicators of success or ways to measure progress in each area. So too when it comes to personal development; now that we have isolated an area (professional career, managerial career, or total human growth), we need to find a way to measure progress.

Growth in these areas, while of interest first of all to the individual himself or herself, is to be agreed upon by both superior and subordinate. The institution wishes to encourage and contribute to this growth, so you will wish to ensure a meeting of the minds between the two of you as to priorities. Hence it is suggested that the individual's *major* personal development needs should be put in writing. The trick is to be as specific as possible. For example, it is not going to help much to tell an individual, "You need to learn to cooperate better with others"; or, "You need to improve your human relations." Instead, try to zero in on one of the three following areas of concern that can be used as indicators to measure progress:

1. Is it some *knowledge* the individual lacks? It could be knowledge of the professional job, knowledge of some management theory, or knowledge of some outside human interest area. For example, when you mention the need to cooperate, are you suggesting the person intellectually does not know what cooperation means, does not identify an occasion when cooperation is called for, does not understand how his/her work ties in with others? If you can demonstrate examples of (a) lack of awareness of the need for cooperation; (b) misun-

derstanding of the type of cooperation called for; or (c) incorrect perception of how far one ought to go in being cooperative, then you enhance the likelihood of corrective action.

2. Is it some *skill* the individual needs to improve? We talk about increasing the level of a skill, acquiring new skills, or sharpening an old skill—all words that suggest there are degrees of an ability or a skill. Again, if you are talking about cooperation, is it a matter of not having the skill of scheduling so as to synchronize adequately one's work with that of others? Is it lack of the skill of negotiating to make the cooperative effort fairly distributed? Is it the lack of an ability to communicate (initiating or receiving) and to coordinate work effectively? Try to recall instances of poor cooperation due to ineptness or poor practice rather than lack of knowledge or awareness.
3. Is it an *attitudinal* concern? Some people have all the knowledge they could want and have demonstrated all the skills they need, but something in their attitude prevents them from using the knowledge and abilities they have. So, when you mention the need to cooperate, you might be suggesting quite deliberate problems. You might mean that the person does not try to do the things he/she knows full well ought to be done, does not want to put out, does not care about how work ties in with that of others. Here you will try to demonstrate instances of a "go-it-alone" attitude, an antagonistic attitude, or any kind of unwillingness to cooperate, rather than lack of knowledge or skill.

Even though interrelated, these three concerns (knowledge, skill, and attitude) ought to be seen as essentially different problems. The point is that clarity about the precise developmental need is necessary in the effort to determine how to measure progress as time goes by. The better job you do in specifying the precise growth need, the more likely you will be able to agree on a remedy for the situation and tell whether things have improved. Managers who are accustomed to defining needs before designing solutions should have no trouble recognizing the importance here of defining developmental needs before moving on to programs of action to meet those needs.

Now it's practice time again.

Question: Identify at least one developmental need you have personally noticed or mentioned to one of your own subordinates. If you have no subordinates, think of a peer. (It's easier to think of someone else before trying to do the same thing for yourself.)

Answer:

Personal Development Activities

Now that you have isolated a specific developmental need for this individual, it will be relatively easy to move on to a suggested course of action to achieve the personal development objective. For here, as in job objectives, results won't happen by themselves: you will have to pursue some action plan to arrive at the desired knowledge, skill, or attitudinal change. You want to work out a meeting of the minds as to the specific steps both of you will take to culminate in the person's growth. Again, specificity is the most important thing in selecting from the publications to be studied, courses to be taken, or any of the possible steps that might be considered, such as the following:

- specific job assignment that will broaden the knowledge or experience of the subordinate, such as temporary appointment, job rotation, vacation fill-in
- reading of specific books, magazines, reports, research publications
- attendance of specific courses in pursuit of special knowledge; seminars, workshops, conferences, and training programs in pursuit of special skills or attitudes
- management development programs, spelling out whether a highly concentrated area of one or two topics is needed or a broad orientation is better
- programmed instruction
- correspondence courses
- association membership; professional group activities at either a local level or a national level
- delivering papers, writing articles, publishing in one way or another
- field trips to other hospitals or organizations
- special assignment, stressing the developmental aspect of such a task
- leadership positions in some organization or cause
- participation in meetings within the hospital that the individual would not otherwise normally attend

- committee work, especially chairing such a group, again stressing the growth aspect of such work
- individual instruction: a one-to-one relationship in which the person might be someone's understudy for a period of time to watch firsthand the knowledge, skill, or attitude needed
- coaching or counseling sessions: planned activities and frequent discussions with the individual to review performance and suggest ways of doing things before mistakes are made or just after projects are completed

From this list it can be seen that attention is being directed at further growth, at future responsibilities, at getting ready for promotion, or for handling present assignments better. These kinds of objectives and the entire process of growth have been neglected in the past because of the tendency to talk about them only in a negative fashion, to resort to them as a sort of punishment or a remedial action.

Question: Work out a plan of action to help your subordinate meet the needs identified in the previous practice box. You might select from the list of Examples 1 to 15 above. Be sure to be precise as to what work, what courses, what readings, and so forth.

Answer:

Commitment from the Organization

Under the MBO philosophy, all objectives involve a mutual commitment. Now that you have identified a course of action for the subordinate to pursue in order to grow, it is time to give some thought as to how you, the manager, can contribute to the developmental process.

Sometimes it has to stop at simply making the recommendations you have been preparing up to this point. At other times you may find it within your power to expend some of the institution's resources to assist the other person in growing. It might be a matter of tuition reimbursement, travel expenses for a workshop, payment for a subscription, spending time in counseling sessions, time off the job to attend some program, arrangements for temporary job reassignment, or the like.

Question: What do you think could be the commitment on the part of you and the organization to assist your subordinate in accomplishing personal development objectives?

Answer:

Evaluation of Personal Development Achievements

You probably just answered that you would provide such things as moral support, advice, and counsel in selecting programs of improvement; time to engage in development activities; financial support to pay for tuition, travel, and other expenses. There must be at least a recognition of the time and effort required and allowances made on the job to compensate for this. How different is the attitude of a supervisor who tells a subordinate, "You want to develop yourself by attending a seminar or other program? Then do it on your own time!"

On the other hand, if the hospital is to pay for classes, meetings, trips, conventions, and the like, there ought to be a policy requiring personnel to explain the nature and purpose of the meeting or workshop when requesting authorization. Too often the agenda is not even known—just the fact that a "professional" meeting will be held on such and such days in such and such a place (and always nice-to-visit places!).

When the developmental activity is over, there ought to be some kind of evaluation as to whether the developmental objective was achieved. Here is the critical point of this whole chapter. When it comes to evaluating personal growth, the question is not, "Did the individual attend the workshop, read the book, go on the trip?" The question ought to be, "Did the workshop, book, or trip result in the individual's achieving the knowledge, skill, or attitudinal change that was the real objective?"

Depending on which of the three your subordinate was after, you will go about evaluating in a different manner. To measure that someone has achieved new knowledge, *tests* will suffice. It could be an academic type test such as given at the conclusion of a course or workshop. It could be just informal feedback over lunch or a cup of coffee upon the individual's return to work. It could be a self-test in that the individual can answer questions, make a presentation, offer a recommendation now based on new knowledge that allows him/her to make the judgment as to whether new knowledge has been acquired.

To measure that a person has acquired or improved some skill, tests will not suffice. Abilities must be *demonstrated.* So upon completion of the developmental activities, your subordinate will wish to demonstrate the skill by actually using it. This is sometimes done at the conclusion of skills-oriented workshops or training sessions right there in the classroom; sometimes there must be follow-up with the individual back on the job.

When it comes to measuring attitudinal change, a third kind of evaluation is called for. You cannot give a person a written test to check on attitudes. Nor can attitudes be demonstrated visibly as skills can. We get at attitudes through *observation of behavior*. It was earlier behavior (what a person said or did) that suggested the need for a change in attitude, and the need was probably brought home by recounting of specific incidents in which undesirable behavior was witnessed. Then observation of subsequent similar incidents must be used to measure that change has taken place. And if it has, the person must be credited with a change in attitude and not presumed to be "superficially different but underneath harboring the same poor attitudes!"

Question: Practice time again. This time see if you can apply the personal development concepts discussed in this chapter to your own need for personal growth.

Answer:

1. I need to grow in the area of: (professional, management, total human growth).

2. I need to acquire this specific knowledge, skill or attitudinal change:

3. I can achieve this growth by means of the following activities, and commit myself to pursue this course of action:

4. I will evaluate my success in accomplishing this personal development in the following manner:

In all three types of personal development measurement, it should be borne in mind that no one is as interested in a person's personal growth as that individual himself/herself. Hence, whether you the manager choose to evaluate personal growth or not, subordinates should be anxious to ascertain whether improvement has taken place or not. That is, they will seek opportunities to evaluate their own personal development. At times this will mean contriving an occasion where new knowledge can be manifested; seeking out opportunities to exercise new skills; deliberately asking to be observed in a role-playing or hypothetical situation, if not in real life, in order to see that attitudes have changed.

SUMMARY

If it is true that no organization can grow any faster than its people, then every individual should be encouraged to include objectives dealing with personal growth. This is most often done on the occasion of the annual review.

Such objectives can deal with growth in a technical/professional career, a management career, or in total human growth. The way to measure that growth takes place is to identify a need for knowledge, skills, or change of attitude. All three can apply to all three classes of personal objectives. The identified needs establish a base. The objective is to satisfy the needs and move to a different level of knowledge, skill, or attitude by some appropriate course of action. This chapter asked you to practice on someone else and on yourself.

Chapter 14

How to Integrate MBO and Quality Assurance

The previous chapter completes our discussion of how to set up a hospitalwide system of operational planning by the participative setting of objectives, both job-related and personal development, at every level of management or supervision. It is a time-consuming and complicated process. Some readers will be thinking about now that they cannot afford the time to set up such a comprehensive system, even if they like it, in the face of other things they *must* do of a related nature. After all, they point out, MBO is a system to see to it that we are accomplishing what we should, and there are other systems or processes that attempt to do the same thing, such as JCAH accreditation visits, Professional Standards Review Organization (PSRO) and other auditing procedures and, most recently, hospitalwide quality assurance (QA) programs. The conclusion sometimes is to go with the systems you have no choice in, and forget the nice, but nonmandated systems like MBO.

The purpose of this chapter is to suggest the integration of MBO and QA by showing how in a sense both are after the same thing under a different name, though one developed out of a need to manage, while the other had its origin in a need to meet regulatory mandates.

BACKGROUND

One of the earmarks of a group of professionals is that it monitors or polices its own activities. Historically, health care professionals have done this through periodic audits—sometimes retrospective, sometimes concurrent. The purpose of these audits in general has been to determine that appropriate work was performed, services were rendered, care was given, "appropriate" meaning usual, customary, or recognized generally by one's colleagues in the profession as called for by the circumstances or conditions of the patient.

With the growth of regulation in the health care industry, regulatory agencies such as the JCAH (for those facilities voluntarily seeking accreditation) and governmental agencies at state and federal levels (for those institutions created by legislative bodies) have mandated that not only physicians and nurses but all health care providers conduct audits of the clinical outputs of their patient care to determine whether or not these outputs are contributing to or helping to maintain acceptable levels of patient care. In many cases the mandate for output audits as opposed to the former process audits was a moot point not considered deserving of much attention or any change in behavior.

Many hospitals decided on their own that if the total hospital were to be true to its mission, then all operating units (clinical and nonclinical) should be expected to make a contribution either to the direct care of the patient as expressed in the mission or to providing an environment conducive to and supportive of that care and service. In this view patient care is described as a continuum on which one service output flows into another until the final outcome of patient care is ultimately achieved. The service outputs that thus make up patient care are provided by clinical as well as nonclinical personnel or units. These service outputs are sometimes called *service elements* and good patient care is therefore achieved by efficient and effective utilization of both clinical and nonclinical personnel and units in the provision of their individual service elements. To review quality of patient care then becomes a matter of reviewing the entire continuum of these service elements.

Attempts to respond to mandated audits on the one hand and voluntary desires to evaluate good patient care from all service units led in time to a proliferation of measures of quality. A listing of these manifold attempts to monitor good care often included:

- PAS (discharge abstracts statistics)
- UR (audit studies by medical staff)
- PSRO (comparative studies by physicians)
- nursing audits
- infection control (through culture exams)
- risk management: incident reports covering
  - medication errors
  - IV errors
  - patient incidents
  - patient property loss
  - procedure errors

- electric shocks, burns, etc.
- safety committee (through hospital rounds)
- operational audits (evaluation/assessment of service elements provided)

Most recently the trend is toward hospitalwide QA programs, receiving their greatest impetus from the JCAH's revised standard on quality for 1980. No single definitive method for complying with this revised standard exists, nor is there a single method of implementing the kind of AQ program now mandated. A review of JCAH literature shows that only general guidelines exist. "There shall be a well-defined, organized, ongoing QA effort designed to demonstrate improvement in patient care."[1] It should be comprehensive or hospitalwide, coordinated with responsibility vested in a single individual, and properly staffed/supported by administration.

As opposed to previous audits that stopped at counting and reporting deficiencies, the new QA program is to be problem-based, which means

- Problems (deficiencies or failures) in the delivery of care are to be identified.
- Appropriate objective assessment strategies are to be selected.
- The problems are to be assessed against criteria to determine the extent and probable causes of the problems.
- Appropriate methods aimed at solving the problems are to be implemented.
- Follow-up is to be done by way of assessment to ensure that the problems have been resolved or reduced.

The centralization of the QA effort through the coordination of a QA office is to ensure a single system of quality assessment in the institution rather than the previous proliferation. The QA effort then will have one location, one staff, one set of rules. An appropriate budget is required to provide sufficient resources to service the hospitalwide effort. A QA multidisciplinary committee is recommended through which all committees and activities concerned with quality of care should report. The person in charge should have high level accountability, that is, should report to the CEO/administrator to emphasize the hospital's commitment to QA.

COMPARISON: QA AND MBO

Before going on to discuss how some hospitals have responded to this new mandate, it is useful to compare these theoretical aspects of a hospitalwide QA program with what the reader now understands to be the important aspects of a viable MBO system.

The most startling word in the revised JCAH standard is the admonition that however a QA program is set up, it is *to demonstrate* improvement in patient care: not be in favor of it, promise it, wave the flag for it—we've been doing that for years—but demonstrate it, for a variety of reasons stemming from the inability of many health care institutions to demonstrate as well as they have waved the flag.

Starting with this amazing similarity in overall orientation, note the following list of similarities:

Item	*MBO*	*QA*
overall orientation	results-oriented	to demonstrate patient care
reports to	CEO	CEO
scope	hospitalwide	hospitalwide
coordinated by	MBO coordinator (staff role)	QA coordinator (staff role)
duration	continual process	ongoing
concerns	routine results	service elements
	problems to be solved	problems to be corrected
	innovative benefits	improvements in care
paper work	written commitment	problems to be documented
plan of attack	action plans	action plans
evaluation	performance review	follow-up (audits)
assessment	indicators & levels	criteria established
priority	support from admin.	support from admin.
for what reason	achieve mission	improve patient care

Is it any wonder then that some have turned to a system of management already existing and flourishing in many hospitals today although it often isn't recognized as QA because it goes by the name of MBO, which, to those not skillful at it, doesn't sound like anything to do with patient care?

WHAT AND WHO OF A QA PROGRAM

According to the National Association of Quality Assurance Professionals, the following is a logical list of initial tasks for the QA initiator in a hospital:[2]

Task No. 1: Identify key actors (who have the power, authority, and influence in the hospital). This is to recognize that a QA program, like any other high priority hospital-wide program, must have the right support. This would include support from the governing body (at least one key designated individual member), the medical staff (especially those who are respected as leaders, both formal and informal), and administration (the CEO directly, if at all possible). These would make up the core group; additional sources of support will depend on the particular institution.

Task No. 2: Identify the ideal. This is a description of the hospital's view of the *best* patient care. It might include the idealistic, the altruistic, the unattainable along with more measurable goals as to the type of patient care desired.

Task No. 3: Examine existing areas. This is an inventory of current QA activities, together with an outline of what they do.

Task No. 4: Compare what you learned in task #2 and task #3. This means a realistic examination of the adequacy of ongoing efforts to ensure realization of desired patient care. QA activities are for the purpose of assessing progress in reaching goals. You may find frustrations, spinning of wheels, duplication of effort, lack of effort, lack of guidance, lack of motivation, some successes certainly, and areas of vacuum.

Task No. 5: Develop your improved QA plan. Using the information gained above, you will consolidate, coordinate, realign, reassign, redefine, and above all renew confidence in an effort to demonstrate improvement in patient care.

The QA plan itself should cover the following:

- the *purpose* of QA and of this plan
- a *chart* (organizational chart or flowchart) to describe the authority, accountability, and communications aspects of the QA program in practice
- the *scope* of the QA activities to ensure their comprehensiveness
- brief description of how the QA program is to be *implemented;* there are four key features:
  1. how problems are to be identified
  2. how priorities are to be set
  3. who has what authority
  4. how to monitor results: who gathers data, who reviews data, who has access to data
- annual *evaluation:* by whom, when, of what, with what consequences

To assist the reader in seeing such a QA program in action and to lay the foundation for the next section that will outline specifics of a QA program integrated into MBO, Exhibits 14-1 and 14-2 are two attempts to set forth a position description for the QA coordinator.

Exhibit 14-1 What and Who of a QA Professional

Education and Experience

1. Direct experience both in management of a hospital unit and in one or more of the QA functions included in the office.
2. A registered nurse or registered records administrator with managerial experience. Additional training in hospital administration or management science would be helpful, or experience in the area in lieu of an RN or RRA.
3. Person must have a sense of the hospitalwide problems and be able to direct problems to appropriate individuals or departments for resolution.

Note: The position may be best filled by a health professional other than an RN or RRA if the necessary background in management and hospital QA are both present.

Line of Authority

The "QA professional" reports in some cases directly to the chief executive of the health facility to ensure the necessary support and resources for accomplishing the objectives of the position/department. In other cases, the QA professional reports to the QA committee. This depends upon the particular QA plan developed.

QA Committee

One central committee to process problem identification data from all QA functions, implement actions, and monitor problems until resolution. Composition of the committee would be dependent upon the QA plan of the hospital.

Responsibilities of a QA Professional

1. Responsible for coordinating and ensuring:
   a. The receiving, collating, and summarizing of all reports on quality assurance and risk management.
   b. The fact that all components of the data collection and control systems are in place and functioning.
   c. The activities of physicians and nonphysicians are used in such a manner that maximum benefit is obtained from the least amount of time possible.
   d. The analysis of problem identification data reported for patterns, relationships, and clusters.
   e. The orientation of all hospital staff is such that they understand the scope, objectives, and procedures of the QA program.
   f. The needed assistance to physician committees is provided for the orientation of the members and other physicians.
2. Other major responsibilities:
   a. Provide resources necessary to the developing of know-how in planning and implementing QA program.
   b. Be instrumental in developing the interest level of administration and medical staff in the QA program.

Exhibit 14-1 continued

c. Be current on all activities related to QA activities and relay these to other interested persons.
d. Be prepared to do the basic drafting of the QA Plan, including forms necessary to document findings.
e. Work closely with medical staff and administrative committees in planning of the program.
f. Provide *continuing inservice* education for personnel and assist with medical staff continuing education.
g. Ensure the *confidentiality* of the QA data.
h. *Supervise all employees* of the QA program.
i. Since a hospital/health care provider may be performing 10, 15, 20, or more QA activities, be responsible for organizing this important function.
j. Screen and solve problems for the QA committee.
k. Other responsibilities as directed or needed by the health care facility or institution.

Source: Robert L. Warner, President, National Association of Quality Assurance Professionals, workshop handout, 1980.

Exhibit 14-2 Position Description for Program Director for Quality Assurance

Appointed by ____________________________
Accountable to ____________________________

Primary Responsibilities

1. Define all activities that relate to a QA program.
2. Identify, integrate, and coordinate existing defined activities into a comprehensive centralized program.
3. Plan, organize, manage, and control activities needed to maintain and enhance an integrated program.

Major Functions

1. Act in a liaison and facilitator capacity to ensure that a comprehensive program is in effect.
   a. Evaluate and advise on composition of a multi-disciplinary QA committee through which all reports on performance from components of the program are received and follow-up action monitored and/or initiated.
   b. Attend meetings of any committee identified as a component of the program.
   c. Assist in the orientation to the program of members of the QA committee of the divisional board.
   d. Ensure that directives of accrediting and regulatory agencies relating to QA are being met.
   e. Participate in liaison with the corporate director of QA for the Sisters of Mercy Health Corporation in creating a model QA program.

Exhibit 14-2 continued

2. Coordinate and analyze data elicited from and produced by departments, committees, and activities relating to QA.
   a. Review, analyze, and summarize audits, reports, and minutes of committees in relation to QA activities.
   b. Prepare and present reports for administration and for meetings of the QA committee of the divisional board.
3. Monitor corrective intervention, follow-up action, and results of action.
   a. Organize and manage a reporting system to identify, analyze, and monitor action and follow-up.
   b. Verify that reevaluation of problem areas identified through audits are performed.

Position Requirements

Academic:	Masters degree preferred
Experience:	Extensive, relevant experience in a health-related discipline to include:
	• collection and interpretation of patient information
	• patient care audits, utilization review, discharge planning
	• membership on patient care and/or medical staff committees
Knowledge of:	• medical and QA terminology
	• literature in the field of QA
	• regulatory and accrediting agency standards and regulations relative to QA, i.e., JCAH, PSRO
Skills in:	• collecting and analyzing data
	• preparing and presenting information in a meaningful manner
	• communicating, orally and in writing
	• developing constructive relationships

Source: Sisters of Mercy Health Corporation, Farmington, MI.

IMPLEMENTING A HOSPITALWIDE QUALITY ASSESSMENT PROGRAM

When the QA professional begins some of the tasks to initiate a QA program, he/she often feels very comfortable analyzing, coordinating, and integrating those QA activities dealing with clinical service areas. Medical audits, nursing audits, tissue committees, UR committees, and the like are familiar territory. But to integrate *all* hospital departments and individuals means going to other sections of that patient care continuum that deal with the hospital environment rather than direct care to the patient, and here the QA professional is usually in strange territory. The need to evaluate the quality of work performed against established criteria in these nonclinical areas has led some to call the entire program *quality assessment* rather than *quality assurance* because of the more narrow scope often read into the latter term. When this is done the term is defined thus:

> *Quality assessment* is the general term for any program that measures the quality of services provided against established criteria.

In a QA plan, the *purpose* of the QA program is "to improve job performance or the services delivered by any individual or department."

An audit of job performance provides data about how the job is being done. The audit may measure outcomes or processes. Outcomes are the results obtained by a particular process. Examples of outcomes are such things as: Does the diabetic patient understand how to control his/her diet? Is the item sterile at the end of the sterilizing process? Has the patient been sent his/her bill?

A process is the *steps* used to achieve the outcome desired. Examples of processes include the classes that are used to instruct the diabetic patient on his/her diet, the sterilizing procedures used to sterilize the item, the flow of paperwork involved in sending a bill to the patient.

The purpose of the audit of either outcome or process is to assess how well each individual/department performs its function. Each should be evaluated based upon the criteria the department sets for itself. Periodic audits are made using those criteria. Data are collected and analyzed. Persons in authority are provided feedback from these data. Problems are identified. Corrective measures are instituted. Follow-up is provided to determine success in correcting the problems. All of the above are documented.

In all programs known to us, participative decision making at each step is a major ingredient for a successful program. The QA operational audit is trying to answer the question, "Are departments meeting their service objectives, or, if not, to what extent are they achieving their stated objectives?" This being the case, the process must take into account those outputs of a department's performance that are considered important to patient care not only in the view of the department itself, but also in the view of the consumers of the department's services. Therefore it is the joint responsibility of those departments that utilize services and those that provide them to identify the critical service elements and once they are identified, to work together to establish acceptable standards of performance to be the criteria for assessing satisfactory performance.

Once service outputs are developed for each department and an effective data collection system is developed and implemented to obtain quantified and objective data, then a manager can ascertain whether or not the stated service outputs are being actually obtained, or if not, to what extent they are being obtained. By quantifying the service element and developing data collection mechanisms, a department is able on a concurrent basis to perform internal self-audits. At the same time this provides readily accessible data for service evaluators to perform external audits on a retrospective basis as well as concurrently.

It is essential in this type of auditing system to develop service outputs that are objective and easily identified in order to obtain a high level of understanding and acceptance from those employees who are performing the service outputs at the department level. It is essential that all workers know what level of output they are working to obtain and maintain and that they are involved in the process of identifying the specific outputs and their levels and measurement.

The intended thrust of the service outputs audit is to totally involve all employees in working together in a team effort to achieve identified critical service elements on a consistent basis. The purpose of the operational audit is to provide managers at the department level a management tool that they can use to determine whether or not their departments are achieving their service objectives. Thus it is an ongoing internal evaluation tool. Periodically (perhaps monthly) an external evaluator performs an external audit using the same criteria to provide an additional outside objective review of a department's attainment of its stated service objectives. A report of this audit can be provided to the department manager's administrative superior and to the CEO so that they can take appropriate administrative action to reward, correct, change, or otherwise respond to the behavior of all in the department.

For purposes of coordination, a QA committee often receives copies of all audit reports and analyses. It is the function of this committee then to review all information, help determine priorities in regard to problem areas needing attention, and to monitor activities related to the accomplishment of recommended and accepted corrective actions, as well as to give guidance in establishing auditing criteria in the first instance. The membership of this committee should reflect the broad range of experience and expertise present in the particular institution/organization. The committee's purpose is to coordinate, to analyze, to recommend, to report findings, to facilitate in numerous ways. Administrative superiors are the ones to take personnel actions.

In making recommendations the committee should prioritize its suggestions so that those that impact patient care the most are addressed first. All recommendations must comply with the standards and criteria established by all external regulatory bodies and internal policies of the institution. When such recommendations impact the operations of the organization financially, they must receive the appropriate administrative approval.

It is essential to resolve issues and concerns that are identified through the audit process. One of the most devastating organizational dynamics that can take place is for the feeling to exist among employees that issues and concerns cannot or do not get resolved. This could lead to organizational apathy, conflict, and confrontation. For this reason, an administrative system for monitoring progress in achieving recommended corrective action must be established to ensure timely closure to all pertinent issues and concerns.

Various methodologies have been devised to reach agreement among department employees and consumers of the department's services about critical service elements and appropriate levels of performance. Sometimes staff persons with management engineering expertise can be useful in facilitating such an agreement. Definitely someone from the QA department should participate in all discussions to determine the departmental criteria and to integrate conclusions into the hospital's overall QA effort by proper recording on forms, dating the decisions, allowing for a trial period, and so forth.

Once the criteria have been established according to some overall schedule that eventually covers the entire hospital, the evaluations should begin. Departmental managers will wish to have their own workers perform internal checks against the standards set for purposes of internal management control. But the QA department should then arrange for regular unannounced external evaluations using the same criteria. Typically a department head from another department, with an employee of that person's choice, will perform the evaluation. Evaluators are assigned at random and will not know which department will be evaluated until the time of the audit. Likewise, the department to be evaluated will not know when its turn will be until the time arrives. Obviously, care must be taken not to cause major interruptions of the smooth flow of a department's work by audits at patently poor times. As a rough rule of thumb, an evaluation should take no more than an hour per department. This means care in the selection of the number of critical service elements and care in choosing indicators of satisfactory performance; usually they deal with quantity, quality, time, or cost considerations.

In most auditing systems of this sort, a method of scoring is worked out, and minimum scoring levels are established as measures of a manager's operating efficiency.

Another element common to most audits of this sort is a requirement that any time a standard is not met (the characteristic of good performance is rejected), an explanation as to why this judgment was made must be included in the report.

A review of Appendixes 14-A to 14-C, which are samples of evaluator sheets for three different kinds of departments, will bring home other aspects in the determination of acceptable standards of performance.

SUMMARY

This chapter has shown the similarity between a hospitalwide MBO program and a hospitalwide quality assurance program. The intent of each is to involve workers in determining criteria for judging satisfactory performance in those areas considered most meaningful in pursuing the mission of the institution and the assigned responsibilities of a given department/individual. Those characteristics of a job done well are used by personnel of the department as well as by outside evaluators to measure performance. When deviations from these standards are detected (problems identified), plans for corrective action are determined and follow-up measures instituted to track improvement. The coordination of this type of activity throughout the hospital is essential, no matter what name is given to the program.

NOTES

1. 1980 JCAH revised standard on Q.A.
2. Robert L. Warner, President, National Association of Quality Assurance Professionals, workshop handout, 1980.

Appendix 14-A

Critical Services Elements: Purchasing Department

Directions: Before beginning your evaluation, look at a calendar and determine the date four, three, two and one *working* day ago. Note these dates on your evaluation sheet. These dates will be needed during your evaluation.

Characteristics	*Acceptance Criteria*
1. Time to Be Assisted by Telephone	1. Call extension 372 during the morning. Reject if not answered by the fourth (4th) ring. When answered go to the next item.
2. Time to Have Telephone Call Returned	2. When the phone is answered, request that any one of the following three people return your call. Reject if the call is not returned by the end of the day. a) ____________________ b) ____________________ c) ____________________
3. Attention to Vendors	3. Proceed to the Materials Management office. Wait in the waiting area until a vendor or salesman asks to see a buyer. Return in twenty (20) minutes. Reject if the vendor is still waiting.
4. Typed Orders	4. Identify yourself to the receptionist as the Quality Evaluator. Ask to see her processed, but untyped, orders. Select five (5) at random. Reject if any are more than two (2) *working* days old.
5. Variance Reports Processing	5. Ask to see __________. Ask __________ for her variance reports. Select five (5) at random. Reject if any are more than four (4) *working* days old as compared with the date stamped on them.
6. Services Orders	6. Ask __________ to see the office equipment service order book. Reject if any orders were not answered within one (1) *working* day.
7. Routine Supply Requisitions (Not Capital Expenditure)	7. Ask one of the buyers for their routine, open purchase requisitions. Select five (5) at random. Reject if any items were not ordered within four (4) working days from the date stamped. The order date is in the lower right hand corner and may or may not be filled in. If it is not filled in, the stamped date must be within the last four (4) working days.
8. Shipping Documents	8. Ask the secretary to accompany you to the receiving area. In the receiving area, ask to see the returned items. Select ten (10) items. Reject if any have been there more than three (3) working days without an acceptable reason.

QUALITY EVALUATION REPORT

Date: ______________
Time of Evaluation: ____________________

CHARACTERISTICS	ACCEPT	REJECT	EXPLANATION FOR REJECT STATUS
1. Time to Be Assisted by Telephone			(Please use the characteristic number)
2. Time to Have Telephone Call Returned			
3. Attention to Vendors			
4. Typed Orders			
5. Variance Reports Processing			
6. Service Orders			
7. Routine Supply Requisitions (Not Capital Expenditure)			
8. Shipping Documents			
9.			
10.			
11.			
12.			
13.			
14.			Continue on reverse side if additional space is needed.

Signature of Evaluators: TOTAL	A =	R =	Add any general comments here:
____________________	SCORE: $\frac{A}{A + R} =$		
____________________			

Department: ____________________
Please return all materials to the Quality Evaluation Office immediately upon completion.

Appendix 14-B

Critical Service Elements: Environmental Services Department

Optimal____________
Acceptable____________
Unacceptable____________

Dept: Environmental Services Location: Ground Floor Effective Date:________

Section I
CRITICAL SERVICE ELEMENTS STANDARD
Patient Room: Go into the assigned rooms and check the following:

1. *Trash Cans:*
   Clean on outside; interior free of gross material. Score %.
   Reason for Rejection: ________

2. *High Dust:*
   Check the following: tops of TVs; shower curtain rod, vents in bathroom, light fixtures. Score %.
   Reason for Rejection: ________

3. *Bathroom:*
   Tub is clean w/o mildew; ceramic tile is clean of soap buildup; no hard water surface rings in toilets; counter tops clean; supplies stocked; toilet tissue, paper towel, soap in dispenser, floor mopped, trash can clean. Score %.
   Reason for Rejection: ________

Room Number	Tally Column Yes	No	Raw Score 0–79	80–89	90–100
			0	1	2

Room Number	Tally Column Yes	Tally Column No	Raw Score 0–79	Raw Score 80–89	Raw Score 90–100
			0	1	2

4. *Wet Mopping:*
   Unacceptable if there is dirt buildup in corners or along edge of baseboards. Ensure that a dirty spot in the tile has not had finish laid over it (take sharp object and scrape through the spot; if the spot does not come up, it has had finish laid over it). Score %.
   Reason for Rejection: ______
   ____
   ____

5. *Glass Areas:*
   Bathroom mirrors and windows must be free from smudges, streaks, and dirt. Score %.
   Reason for Rejection: ______
   ____
   ____

6. *Carpets:*
   Carpets must be free from gross soiled areas; must appear to have been vacuumed within the last 16 hours. Score %.
   Reason for Rejection: ______
   ____
   ____

7. *Trash:*
   Look in service closets on the floors specified; unacceptable if any of the following is evident: trash on the floor or shelves seem unorganized. Score %.
   Reason for Rejection: ______
   ____

	Room Number	Tally Column Yes	Tally Column No	Raw Score 0–79	Raw Score 80–89	Raw Score 90–100
				0	1	2
8. *Walls:* Randomly select 6 areas and check the walls around the light switch, door jams, in sills and walls for accumulation of dirt. Score %. Reason for Rejection: ______						
9. *Vinyl Floor Areas:* Randomly select 6 vinyl tile areas on the assigned floors. An area is unacceptable if any one of the following is evident: buildup of dirt on baseboards, in corners or along the edges of the baseboard. When looking at corridors, check to see if there is a high gloss to the tile. Score %. Reason for Rejection: ______						
10. *Carpets:* Randomly select 6 rooms in the nonpatient areas; select one corridor; check carpet for gross contaminants; look in offices to see if vacuumed. Score %. Reason for Rejection: ______						
Subtotal						
Score × 1.25						

Additional Comments:

Optimal ____________
Acceptable__________
Unacceptable________

Dept: Environmental Services Location: Ground Floor Effective Date: ________

Section II *CRITICAL SERVICE ELEMENTS*	Room Number	Tally Column Yes	No	Raw Score 0–79	80–89	90–100
1. *Personnel Appearance:* An employee shall be in blue uniform. Name tag should be present. 0/2				0	1	2
2. *Housekeeping Request:* Check with any department; ask if they have requested any services through the Environmental Services Office; then check telephone logs at the secretary's desk. If request is not logged, and given to appropriate personnel, score unacceptable.						
3. *Fire Safety:* Ask 6 employees						
R—Remove patient						
A—Alarm; call 1444 and report location						
C—Contain. Seal off, shut windows & doors; turn off electricity and oxygen.						
E—Extinguish or evacuate. 0/2						
4. *Carts and Equipment:* Check equipment for good repair, neatness, clean, no clutter. 0/2						
5. *Policy and Procedure Book:* Employee must retrieve Policy & Procedure Books—Hospital and Department—within 5 minutes. Check to ensure a usable index. Ensure all procedures are on proper form, with policy code number and page number required. 0/2						
Subscore						
Total Score						
Total Score ÷ 30						

Additional Comments:

Appendix 14-C
Critical Service Elements: Radiology

Optimal ____________
Acceptable ____________
Unacceptable ____________

Dept: Radiology/Inpatient Location: 1st. Floor Effective Date: ________

Section I
CRITICAL SERVICE ELEMENTS

1. *Emergency Cart:*
   Ask a technician in the department where the emergency cart is kept. Verify that the cart is there. Unacceptable if:
   A. Technician does not know.
   B. Cart is not there.
   Ask a technician the procedure for checking the cart. Unacceptable if:
   A. He/she does not show the supply list.
   B. He/she does not say to check for the white locks; if the box is locked, it is stocked.
   Ask a technician to identify the supply list check sheet. Unacceptable if:
   A. He/she cannot do so in 3 minutes.
   B. The sheet has not been signed at least once a day for the past month.
   Ask any technician the procedure for restocking the cart after use. Unacceptable if he/she does not say, "SRC card attached to box and both returned to the appropriate department and exchanged with a properly stocked box." Score 0/2
2. *X-Ray Availability:*
   Randomly select and record the name and number of 5 patients x-rayed within the past 3 months using receptionist's log. Folders

Room Number	Tally Column Yes	Tally Column No	Raw Score 0–79	Raw Score 80–89	Raw Score 90–100
			0	1	2

Optimal__________
Acceptable__________
Unacceptable________

Dept: Radiology/Inpatient Location: 1st. Floor Effective Date:________

Section I
CRITICAL SERVICE ELEMENTS

Room Number	Tally Column Yes	Tally Column No	Raw Score 0–79	Raw Score 80–89	Raw Score 90–100
			0	1	2

should be located within 10 minutes unless charts are listed in the loan book. Score %.

3. *Response Time/E.R. Department*
   From the time requested to the time responded should not exceed 15 minutes. Check the log for the last 24-hour period to determine how many requests met the criteria. Score percentage.
4. *Procedure Completed Time/ E.R. Department:*
   Procedure completed time for entire process should not exceed 45 minutes. Check log for the last 24-hour period to determine how many requests met the criteria. Score %.
5. *Reports/E.R. Department:*
   Check exceptions log kept by the transcriptionist for a one-week period. X-ray report must have the following: E.R. physician's interpretation, his initials, or signature. If there is no more than one per day that does not meet standard and the weekly average is less than one per day, score 2; if there are 5 during the reporting period (no more than one per day), score Acceptable (1 point); if there is more than one per day or 5 during the period, score Unacceptable (0 points).

Optimal__________
Acceptable__________
Unacceptable__________

Dept: Radiology/Inpătient Location: 1st. Floor Effective Date:________

Section I
CRITICAL SERVICE ELEMENTS

Room Number	Tally Column Yes	No	Raw Score 0–79	80–89	90–100
			0	1	2

6. *Film Return:*
   E.R. films must be returned to the X-ray Department within 4 hours. Check the log to see how many met criteria. Score %.
7. *Report Time:*
   From the log book at the receptionist's desk, select the names, room numbers, and exams of 10 patients from two days prior. Proceed to the floor. X-ray reports should be on the chart with the exception of exams performed from Saturday noon to Monday 7:00 A.M. Score percentage.
8. *Transport Slips:*
   A. Check 5 transport slips for the day. Each must be initialed by the nursing unit indicating that they know the patient left the unit. Score %.
9. *Equipment Performance and Service:*
   Ask for the equipment performance and service record. Unacceptable if:
   A. It cannot be located.
   B. There is no entry for the past five days.
   C. A problem reported over 24 hours ago has not been corrected.
   0/2

Optimal__________
Acceptable__________
Unacceptable__________

Dept: Radiology/Inpatient Location: 1st. Floor Effective Date:_______

Section I *CRITICAL SERVICE ELEMENTS*	Room Number	Tally Column Yes	No	Raw Score 0–79	80–89	90–100
				0	1	2
10. *Doctor's Copies of Reports:* Check file box in transcription area. If there are two or more reports that are not in the doctor's box by 12 noon of the day following the exam, score "0"; if there is one, score "1"; if there is none, score "2."						
Subtotal						
Score × 1.25						

Part IV

The Budgeting and Evaluating Parts of MBO

Chapter 15

How to Budget for Objectives

If MBO is a total system of management as posited in Chapter 1, you are not through with MBO just because you have negotiated meaningful, measurable, and communicable objectives as recommended in the previous parts of this book. You have planned the results you wish to achieve, and in some cases (for the nonroutine objectives) you have discussed briefly your proposed action plans and associated costs in terms of time, money, and energy.

It is now time to integrate that plan with the other institutional control systems set up to conserve resources and encourage cost-effectiveness. This is, of course, the function of the budget. In a results-oriented system of management the budget is to provide the inputs necessary to produce the desired outputs.

This requires a shift in the mentality of the typical manager with regard to the budgeting process. In most cases, managers develop their budgets by using the current level of operations as an established base. Given this base, they then itemize only desired increases, thus looking at only a small fraction of the final budget dollars. This approach does not require a detailed review of ongoing operations and expenditure levels. It might be called *incremental budgeting*.

A newer approach called *zero-based budgeting* has a very different purpose. It is a management tool that provides a systematic way to evaluate operations and programs and provides the potential of shifting resources into what are considered to be the highest priority programs. Rather than being a way of reducing a manager's allocation of finances, this approach has the following psychological advantages:

- Managers throughout the organization have an opportunity to recommend how money should be spent.
- Managers have a chance to evaluate their programs and to change their operations to improve efficiency and effectiveness.

- High priority new programs can be funded by improving cost performance or by reducing or eliminating current programs with lower priorities. These priorities are established by managers throughout the entire organization.
- Participation by managers throughout the organization will improve communications and discussions of key issues and problems for the good of all.

The purpose of this chapter is to outline a practical method of tying the budget to the objectives of a manager, using the principles of zero-based budgeting.

DECISION PACKAGES

A *decision package* identifies a discrete activity or operation (e.g., a department) for management evaluation and comparison with other activities (departments). In this chapter the forms used to illustrate this process are thus called "activity decision packages." The activity decision package is the building block of the zero-based budgeting process. The purpose of the activity decision package is to allow an evaluation of each activity or operation that will include:

- proposed means of performing the activity
- costs and benefits
- workload and performance measures
- implications of not funding the activity
- alternative means of accomplishing activity objectives

An important aspect of developing decision packages is the development of meaningful alternatives. Two types of alternatives should be considered in developing activity decision packages:

1. Alternative methods of performing the same activity. After consideration of various alternatives, the best alternative is chosen and the others are discarded. Only one decision package is prepared for an activity. It shows the recommended method of performing the function and identifies the alternative ways considered, giving a brief explanation of why they were not chosen. If an alternative to the current method of "doing business" is chosen, the recommended way should be shown in the decision package with the current way

shown as an alternative, along with the reason for rejecting it for the future.

2. Different levels of effort for performing the activity, along with different levels of funding that would be called for. This analysis identifies alternative amounts of budget dollars for a specific activity. A base level (minimum level of work) will be established, and additional levels identified as alternatives to be considered in the decision package.

The Base Level

The base level is what we have been considering minimum acceptable level of performance in that it takes this base level of activity/funding to produce the minimum level of results. As a rule, the base level will be below the current level of effort/funding. It will attempt to identify "that critical level of effort, below which the activity should be discontinued because it loses its viability or effectiveness." The relation between all these becomes clear if we recall the systems diagram discussed in Chapter 1:

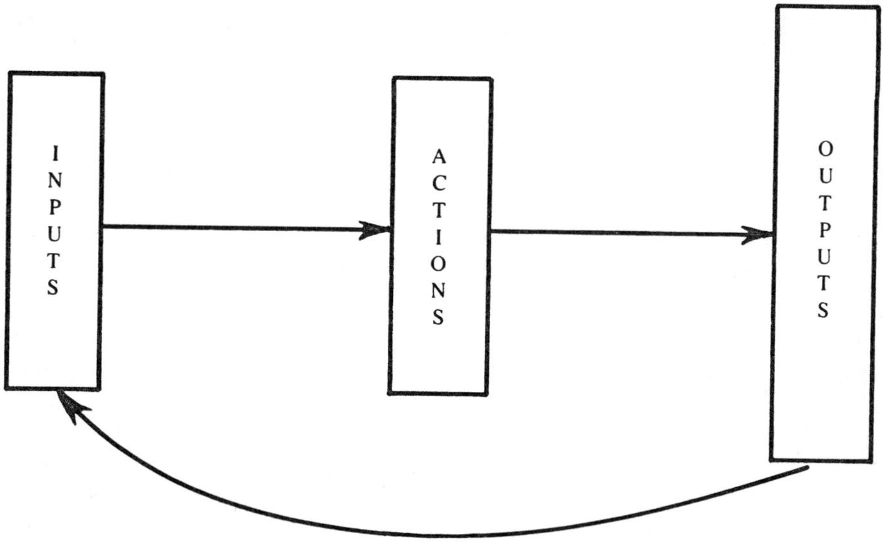

To produce a minimum level of results (outputs) requires a certain minimum level of activity (actions), which in turn calls for a minimum level of funding (inputs). Since minimum acceptable results is defined as that level below which performance will be unsatisfactory, then effort below that same level must be what we are calling the base: that is, below which the activity is no longer viable/productive. That in turn defines the base level of budgeting, so that if funds are not available at least for that level, the program should be abandoned as unlikely to produce meaningful results. This will prevent expenditure of money and effort that is fruitless; it also prevents a superior from expecting high levels of results without providing the necessary funding for needed activities to produce those levels of results.

There are several considerations that can guide managers in defining the base level:

1. The base level may reduce the amount of service provided by each activity but should attack the most serious problems in that area.
2. The base level may not permit complete achievement (expected average and maximum probable levels of objectives) and that is recognized ahead of time.
3. In identifying the base level, the activity (department) manager is not necessarily recommending that the activity be funded at the base level and may identify additional levels that would increase the funding well in excess of the current level. The base level merely identifies one alternative and identifies what could be produced at that level, with the consequences of not funding at the minimum level, or additional levels, clearly stated on the decision package, as they were on the objective sheet.

Note: The additional levels may be of any size, but typically are geared to producing the results already specified as expected average and maximum probable results. They generally are larger than the base package but not so large that the very size precludes the possibility of funding (a very large add-on usually indicates a separately identifiable activity for which a separate decision package should be prepared).

Ranking of Decision Packages (Setting Priorities)

Following the preparation of decision packages for all activities in their organizations, managers rank each level of all packages in priority order using a second form called "Summary of Decision Package Ranking." Frequently a departmental manager will have only one decision package and therefore will not need to do any ranking.

The base level of each package must be ranked higher than the add-on levels of that package. However, add-on levels of one package may be ranked higher than the base levels of other packages. Furthermore, new activities may be ranked higher than current activities.

In ranking, managers should not waste time trying to determine which of two activity levels is first priority and which is second when they can reasonably assume funding of both. Efforts should be concentrated on the order of those packages whose priorities are lower, and therefore funding less certain.

The manager's ranking, as well as the decision packages themselves, are forwarded up the administrative chain to be used successively in consolidating rankings.

Instructions for Completing Activity Decision Package Form

Exhibit 15-1 is a two-page form for presenting the zero-based budgeting analysis for each activity (department). Each section on the form should be complete in itself, with no sentences carrying over onto additional pages. This limitation is intentional. It requires a very concise presentation of the request for funds. This form will usually serve as the entire presentation of each activity (department); however, it may be accompanied by backup material and analysis documents if necessary.

This is intended to be a budget to cover operational activities to achieve operational objectives. As such it will usually include items typically placed on both "expense budgets" and "capital expenditure budgets." To keep this form brief, whenever a decision package contains a request for capital outlay, it does not replace the customary, more detailed justification in the capital expenditure budgeting process.

1. *Account Name:* Title of the account/department through which funding for this activity will be made. An activity decision package should be defined so that it is not funded by more than one account. However, an account (department) may have several decision packages. The fact that funding has become available for a certain activity from a specific source (e.g. the hospital auxiliary, a foundation, a grant) is no reason to "charge" the funds to be spent to those sources. They provide income; here we're concerned with where funds are spent.
2. *Account Number:* The accounting number of the above account, as assigned by the accounting department.
3. *Package Number:* A unique number arbitrarily assigned by the account manager to each activity decision package submitted. It is suggested that the decision packages be numbered consecutively, beginning with the number *1*, with the numbers assigned *after* prioritization has been accomplished. (Some departments will have only one decision package.)

4. *Activity Name:* Descriptive title of the activity that is the subject of the activity package. The word *activity* is here used more in the sense of function or program than in the sense of a single action. On a nursing unit, it will be something like "Direct Patient Care" and will subsume most of the day-to-day objectives. Other nursing unit activities might be "Training of Staff" or "Pilot Program on Primary Care," and the like. In other units there will be activities such as "Special Radiological Procedures," "Delivering Meals to Patients," "Admitting Patients as Inpatients," "Cleaning Patient Rooms." The reader will notice a close connection between this wording and what we called KRAs in earlier chapters: close but not quite identical. Sometimes there are activities that are undertaken

Exhibit 15-1 Activity Decision Package

(1) Account Name		(2) Acct. No.	(3) Pkg. #	(4) Activity Name	
(5) Description of This Activity					
(6) Objectives for This Activity					
KRA	*Indicators*	*Current Yr.*	*Minimum Acceptable*	*Expected Average*	*Maximum Probable*
(7) Cost/Funding Requested [from (12)]					
(8) Method of Performing Activity at Minimum (Base) Level			(9) Implications of Not Funding at This Level		
Method of Performing Activity at Average Level			Implications of Not Funding at This Level		
Method of Performing Activity at Maximum Level			Implications of Not Funding at This Level		
(10) Submitted by			(11) Date		

Exhibit 15-1 continued

(1) Account Name	(2) Acct. No.	(3) Pkg. #	(4) Activity Name	
(12) Cost details	*Current Year*	*Minimum Acceptable*	*Expected Average*	*Maximum Probable*
a. Dept operation Wages (hourly) Travel Maintenance/oper. Supplies Capital outlay Computer svc. Subtotal: b. Salary budget Admin. Professional Nonprofessional Subtotal: Totals				
(13) Manpower (title) Totals	*FTE*	*FTE*	*FTE*	*FTE*
(14) Alternative Methods of Accomplishing This Activity				

as a specific means to solve a problem, but they are not the only work undertaken to provide the results included therein. For example, an activity might be "Risk Management Program," undertaken to reduce patient accidents, employee injuries, and other undesirable results. But these latter are also part of larger KRAs such as "patient care."

5. *Description of This Activity:* A prose version of the purpose or general intent of the work to be performed or explanation in layman's language of the reason behind the technical or professional work to be done.
6. *Objectives for This Activity:* A direct steal from the previously completed objective worksheets, whether routine, problem-solving, or innovative, in that the measures of workload/performance come

from the negotiated objectives. Revenue-producing departments must include somewhere in the total of their activity decision packages an estimate of forecast revenue as one of the measures of their performance. For example, the activity "Special Radiological Procedures" will have one KRA or indicator of success called "revenue generated."

7. *Cost/Funding Requested:* Four different dollar amounts are expected. Under "Current Year" put down the budgeted amount for this activity, not the actual-to-date or year-end projection, though these should be part of any discussion of the budget if materially different from the budgeted amount.

   Under "Minimum Acceptable" put down the base level as discussed in the previous section of this chapter. Under "Expected Average" and "Maximum Probable" put the dollar amounts projected to underwrite the activity levels needed to bring about the results shown in the respective column.
8. *Method of Performing Activity at:* Description of detailed actions to be taken to achieve the objectives. *How* is the work to be performed, the program to be carried out, the results to be achieved? It is understood that to produce successively better results as you move from minimum to maximum columns, actions in lower level columns will be carried over and added to in subsequent columns, so only discuss the "add-on" work.
9. *Implications of Not Funding at This Level:* Explanation of impact on the patient, the department, or the institution if funding is not provided at this level. It goes without saying that comments should be specific here. It will do no good to write: "If funding not received, poor patient care will result."
10. *Submitted by:* This is the name of the account manager, the person who has budgeting responsibility for the account. In some hospitals this will mean no lower than a department manager if supervisory personnel within the department do not have budgeting responsibilities. In such a case the department head would be the one to "defend" the budget, after negotiating the objectives at lower levels.
11. *Date:* The date on which the activity decision package was prioritized along with others in the same account area and forwarded to higher level of management.
12. *Cost Details:* Costs required to support the activity at each level in each of the categories specified. Each column is cumulative (inclusive of dollar amounts) for the same line item in previous columns (not counting the present year). The totals will be carried back to item 7.

The budget of an account that has more than one activity decision package must be allocated among all of its packages, even if such an apportionment was not intended or rigorously adhered to. The reason is that the sum total of an account's budget for the current year will be compared with the sum total of all the account's decision packages for the next year. Admittedly, some items (supplies, salaries) will be arbitrarily divided among several activities in the account (department).

13. *Manpower:* Full time equivalents (FTEs) of personnel required in each classification at each level of activity. The same comments as mentioned under item 12 above apply here.
14. *Alternative Methods of Accomplishing This Activity:* Description of realistic alternatives to the recommended methods of performing the activity, the reasons for rejection, and the estimated costs. If the alternatives do not apply to all levels, indicate to which levels they do apply. A statement of totally unrealistic alternatives does not really bolster the request for funding; it sometimes shows that the account manager has not done the required homework before deciding on this approach, and it may result in a denial or delay.

Exhibit 15-2 is an example of this same two-page form as it might be completed for a rather simple activity.

Instructions for Summary of Decision-Package Ranking

Exhibit 15-3 is a form for the ranking of all levels of all the decision packages. Note that an account with only one activity decision package will still have a summary page in order to list the ranking of the three levels on the one activity.

1. *Account Name:* Same as above.
2. *Account Number:* Same as above.
3. *Summary Submitted by:* Name of account manager, who will stand ready to "defend" the account's budget request.
4. *Summary Submitted to:* The next level manager who must assimilate this budget request into all others of those reporting to him/her and rank the packages of all those account managers into a consolidated whole.
5. *New Rank:* This is a workspace for the manager who receives this summary and must accumulate and rank these packages and levels with others submitted by other managers.

Exhibit 15-2 Activity Decision Package

(1) Account Name Grounds Maintenance	(2) Acct. No. 1234	(3) Pkg. # 1	(4) Activity Name Mowing the Lawn

(5) Description of This Activity
This hospital has 25 acres of lawn, not including flower beds or roadways. It must be mowed for fire safety and appearance.

(6) Objectives for This Activity

KRA	*Indicators*	*Current Yr*	*Minimum Acceptable*	*Expected Average*	*Maximum Probable*
Lawn care	Max grass height	6 in.	12 in.	6 in.	2 in.
	Green months	4 mos.	4 mos.	4 mos.	8 mos.
	Cost per acre	$600	$340	$660	$1600
(7) Cost/Funding Requested [from (12)]		$15,000	$8,500	$16,500	$40,000

(8) Method of Performing Activity at Minimum (Base) Level	(9) Implications of Not Funding at This Level
Mow monthly during grass-growing season (Mar–Oct), to keep height within fire department safety standard of 12 in. maximum.	If this mowing is not performed, grass will grow beyond standard. We would invite citations as well as complaints from neighbors. Tall grass easily catches debris and becomes unsightly quickly.
Method of Performing Activity at Average Level Increase mowing to biweekly intervals to reduce height of grass. This is approximately current level.	Implications of Not Funding at This Level At the base-level funding, only fire standards have been met. Appearance has been neglected.
Method of Performing Activity at Maximum Level Mow weekly. Begin supplementary irrigation and fertilization (capital expense for fertilizer & irrigation system).	Implications of Not Funding at This Level Without this level the lawn will burn/die 8 months of year.
(10) Submitted by G. Patton	(11) Date / /

Exhibit 15-2 continued

(1) Account Name Grounds Maintenance	(2) Acct. No. 1234	(3) Pkg. # 1	(4) Activity Name Mowing the Lawn	
(12) Cost Details	*Current Year*	*Minimum Acceptable*	*Expected Average*	*Maximum Probable*
a. Dept Operation				
Wages (hourly)	$ 500		$ 500	$ 1000
Travel				
Maintenance/oper.	2500	$2500	4000	6000
Supplies				
Capital outlay				12,000
Computer svc.				
Subtotal:	3000	2500	4500	19,000
b. Salary budget				
Admin.	12,000	6000	12,000	21,000
Professional				
Nonprofessional	12,000	6000	12,000	21,000
Subtotal:	12,000	6000	12,000	21,000
Totals	15,000	8500	16,500	40,000
(13) Manpower (title)	FTE	FTE	FTE	FTE
Groundskeeper	2.0	1.0	2.0	3.5
Totals				
(14) Alternative Methods of Accomplishing This Activity Contract mowing: $10,000 to cut monthly (applies to base level only)				

Exhibit 15-3 Summary of Decision-Package Ranking

(1) Account Name		(2) Account No.		(3) Submitted by:	(4) Submitted to:	
(5) New Rank	(6) Pkg No.	(7) Level	(8) Activity Name	(9) Rank	(10) Current Budget	(11) Funding Requested

6. *Package No.:* The package number for the activity and its level itemized on that line. This is only in case additional information might be useful later.
7. *Level:* The level for the activity whose budget request will be listed on this line. There will usually be three different levels recorded on this summary sheet, though sometimes the objective in question will not admit of more than one level. For example, if the decision package concerns "reaccreditation visit" or "hiring a horticulturist," there may not be a range of possible outcomes.
8. *Activity Name:* Copied verbatim from the decision package.
9. *Rank:* This is the rank of the packages and levels according to the submitting manager.
10. *Current Budget:* As indicated, this is the amount budgeted for this level of activity, taken from the decision package form.
11. *Funding Requested:* These are the amounts taken from the various levels of activities on the decision packages (totals only as indicated in item 7 of that form).

Exhibit 15-4 is an example of this same form as it might appear for the account manager whose decision package was earlier illustrated.

Exhibit 15-4 Summary of Decision-Package Ranking

(1) Account Name Ground Maintenance		(2) Account No. 1234		(3) Submitted by: G. Patton		(4) Submitted to: E. Fauver
(5) New Rank	(6) Pkg No.	(7) Level	(8) Activity Name	(9) Rank	(10) Current Budget	(11) Funding Requested
	1	1	Mowing the lawn	1	$15,000	$ 8,500
	1	2	Mowing the lawn	2	15,000	16,500
	2	1	Gardens/landscape	3	6,000	4,000
	3	1	Hire horticulturist	4	0	5,000
	1	3	Mowing the lawn	5	15,000	23,500
	2	2	Gardens/landscape	6	6,000	8,000

[Notes: Three decision packages are submitted for Account No. 1234. Mowing the lawn had 3 possible levels; gardens/landscaping had only 2 levels; hire horticulturist had 1.

Mr. Fauver will prepare a summary page like this one, to include these and all accounts reporting directly to him.

There are no totals on this summary; each line is to be read in its own right.]

TIMING OF THE BUDGETARY PROCESS

As can be seen from the forms for a decision package, the various funding levels are dependent upon the minimum, average, and maximum results negotiated as objectives for a given manager. This means that determination of the objectives must precede computation of related budget amounts.

At the same time, it is difficult to plan objective levels, and do so with a great deal of confidence in the numbers, without a reasonably accurate estimate of what the current year's performance will be: that is, some months' experience "under your belt."

Since the budgeting process takes considerable time as an annual series of events, this means it has to start soon enough before the next fiscal year to pass through all the necessary decision points, yet late enough during the current fiscal year to have meaningful estimates. A schedule should therefore be worked out that dovetails the objective-negotiating process with the budgeting process so that one starts at about the same time as the other. Timing on these things is always dependent upon deadlines imposed by local boards, corporate offices, funding bodies, and the like, but they can often be persuaded to modify their dates if good reasoning is given.

A workable schedule, assuming a fiscal year corresponding to the calendar year, could look like the following:

Date	*Objectives*	*Budget*
1. mid-May (1st qtr complete; ½ of 2nd qtr over)	Administrative retreat to draft hospitalwide objectives for next fiscal year	Capital expenditure forms distributed for next fiscal year
2. mid-June	Hospital objectives approved by board and distributed	Depts complete capital expenditure forms based on hospital priorities
3. mid-July (2 qtrs are complete)	Asst administrators draft objectives with their dept heads	Capital expenditures approved by board
4. 1st week of August	Asst administrators negotiate objectives with exec director	Decision package forms distributed
5. mid-August	Dept heads draft objectives with their supervisors	Asst administrators complete decision pkgs and hold them
6. 1st week of Sept	Dept heads negotiate objectives with assts	

Date	*Objectives*	*Budget*
7. mid-Sept. (almost 3 qtrs complete)	Supervisors draft their objectives	Dept heads complete decision pkgs and hold them
8. 1st week of October	Supervisors negotiate objectives with dept heads	
9. mid-Oct	MBO coordinator compiles master list of all objectives	Supervisors complete decision pkgs and summary and submit to dept heads
10. late Oct		Dept heads summarize decision pkgs and submit to assts
11. 1st week of November		Assts summarize decision pkgs and submit to exec director
12. mid-Nov (3 qtrs complete; ½ of 4th qtr over)		Budget coordinator has total budget ready for board
13. month of December	Renegotiation of any objectives because of casualties in budgeting approval	Rankings on summary sheets finalized and discussed

SUMMARY

When you manage by objectives, you decide the results you intend to make happen, then determine the appropriate work that must be done to achieve those results; only then do you finalize budgeting requirements to do the work that will achieve those results. This chapter has explained and exemplified procedures that can integrate the objective-setting process and the budgeting process in such a way that objectives are finalized before budgets are finalized. Because availability of large capital sums is of particular importance in being able to set objectives, the scheduling of events has kept capital budgeting in advance of rash negotiation both of objectives and operational budgets.

Chapter 16

How to Monitor Progress toward Objectives

You wouldn't think much of an airplane pilot who filed a flight plan and then flew off into the friendly skies in a direction or pattern of directions that had no similarity to that plan. Nor would you think much of a homemaker who worked out a detailed budget to provide for all the needs of the members of the household and then went on a buying splurge that bought a lot of luxuries with funds carefully set aside for essentials. Neither should you think much of a manager who negotiates a carefully thought out list of objectives, supported by budgetary resources, and then operates a unit of the hospital without much regard to either of these documented plans.

In our experience, the main reason, by far, that MBO does not achieve the success it could in many organizations is lack of use of objectives in carrying on day-to-day operations. It seems too easy to go from one crisis to another, from one interruption to another, from one meeting to another, just letting things happen instead of making things happen: that is, with the results negotiated earlier. One of the principal reasons for implementing MBO in the first place is usually a desire to get out of the crisis mode of operation. Yet it is so easy to slip back into that mode and then say rather smugly, "Well, I guess those objectives looked nice on paper, but they don't seem to have anything to do with my unit, because I've managed to run it for another year without much reference to those objectives!"

Such a comment begs the question. Did you really run the unit for another year, or did it run you for another year? And for how many years can this continue before you (or someone higher up) find the place in a shambles due to just letting things slide along? If we don't follow the flight plan we file, we may arrive at our destination, but only by sheer luck, and who knows at what peril to those around us? If we don't live according to the family budget, we may not starve to death, but only if someone bails us out, or we go into debt for the rest of our lives, or we eke out a subsistence level existence. So in running a unit: it may still be existing after another year, but who knows how much better our service could have been or how fewer headaches we could have caused others around us if we had only followed our plan?

When it comes to using objectives for their intended purpose, that is, to monitor progress toward desired results, there are not a lot of "how to's." The most important thing is the determination to operate according to the agreed-upon objectives. So the most important question might be "How to follow through on the resolution to use the objectives?" Just having the objectives isn't really worth anything. It is *managing* by objectives that counts.

There are a few techniques we have found useful in the day-to-day use of objectives throughout the period of operations. This chapter will discuss in turn: techniques of reporting, methods to keep vital and current, ways to follow up, and examples of getting a shot-in-the-arm.

REPORTING TECHNIQUES

How to measure progress in reaching objectives ought to mean in the first instance use of objectives as a method of measuring progress as time goes by. MBO is the only system of management we know in which individuals have a method of evaluating their own performance during the period of operations. We suggest the following techniques to assist managers at any level in using objectives as a kind of daily performance review.

1. Monthly reports. Most hospitals have some kind of routine reporting system in which most of the larger departments in particular find an opportunity to report on such things as volume of units of service, revenue, and status of major items such as delinquent charts, waiting lists for admission, and the like. Where such a monthly operational report is already in use, it can be quite simple to add a section entitled "Report on Progress Toward Objectives." Since for the most part such operational reports are usually statistics, the additional section would be expected to call mainly for statistical information to be compared with similar information on the list of objectives. Such a comparison should consider actual performance to date against where one has a right to expect to be in relation to a year's objectives, and not automatically to one-twelfth of a year's results, due to whatever fluctuation there might be in the course of a year attributable to cyclical variations.

2. Quarterly reports. Even smaller units for which monthly reports are not appropriate should have a requirement to submit a quarterly report of progress toward negotiated objectives. Three months is a large piece of a year's operations, and if progress is not measured after such a large segment of time, it may become too late to make any corrections if they are needed. Three months is also a considerable portion of a year's expenditure of energy, and if recognition of results achieved in such a long block of time is not forthcoming, a person's motivation could wane substantially.

   In both monthly reports and quarterly reports, it is recommended that the exception principle be used. That is to say, only those things for which some results were expected by that time in the progress of the year should be commented upon. It wastes everyone's time and energy to have reports saying: "Objective #3: No results were expected until June of this year, and since it is only March no results have yet been achieved."

   The use of quarterly reports as review sessions will be discussed under the next subheading, Keeping Current.
3. Management Information System (MIS). Very often an operating department will not be in a position to report on its own progress in achieving results: it may need data fed back to it from the accounting department, the computer services department, or some other service unit (personnel, etc.) that has the responsibility to keep statistics. It has been mentioned several times in this book that implicit in putting something down as an indicator of success in an objective is a commitment to keep the records that will allow monitoring of progress. This means that when managers negotiate objectives with their administrative superiors, they must have some idea as to how they will get the information they need to keep on top of the objective. At times the keeper/distributor of such information is indicated on overall hospital objectives under the "Responsibility" column. Other times it is a matter of the manager setting up or requesting the record-keeping mechanism. *Lack of ability to report on progress due to lack of information later* is without doubt the most frequent cause of MBO systems losing their initial excitement/support.

   Sometimes the solution is setting up a complete MIS on computer. Sometimes it is a less sophisticated system of providing the same information through staff offices such as accounting. Sometimes management engineers are of assistance in setting up standards and recording mechanisms. Sometimes staff personnel in a QA department furnish the statistics, based on the responsibility to coordinate evaluators as discussed in Chapter 14.

Operating units are customarily too busy doing the work to have the time to keep the records, even when they want to, so this must be kept in mind in choosing the indicators of success and in allocating resources in staff offices. The latter are advised to check with unit managers to find out what information they want kept rather than reporting information that won't be used.

KEEPING CURRENT

For managers to be able to manage by their lists of objectives, the objectives must have relevance to day-to-day requirements of the job. It was for this reason that so much emphasis was placed earlier on including "routine" objectives in the list. For the same reason, the list must be made to continue to refer to the ongoing work of the unit, that is, to continue to be current. In this manner the list is truly a vital document, at all times a roadmap for steering the group's activities. Just as "there is nothing older than yesterday's news," so there is nothing so useless to a manager than a list of objectives that made sense on the day it was negotiated but was allowed to become obsolete. We recommend the following methods of keeping objectives meaningful.

1. Quarterly updates. The quarterly report was mentioned in the preceding section. That written report should serve as the basis for a face-to-face meeting between the same two people who negotiated the objectives for the purpose of updating the list. Objectives are not straitjackets. A commitment to achieve certain results is valid only as long as the results in question are still meaningful, measurable, and realistic. If, for any reason, the two parties to the original managerial contract feel that an objective is no longer valid, it ought to be renegotiated. Notice it takes both parties to renegotiate: neither one should be able to abrogate the contract unilaterally.

   Some objectives will be found to be unrealistic in the levels of achievement originally sought. Other times it will be found that an indicator of success really doesn't measure what it was supposed to, or the information turns out not to be available, or perhaps it was just a meaningless indicator now that an alternative has been thought of. In some cases it will be found that a result is happening whether it was included on the list or not (as opposed to something we're trying to *make* happen). Sometimes newer objectives have been thought of that change the priority of something on the list. Once in a while an objective will have been accomplished since the last meeting of the two negotiators. All of these are occasions for changing, deleting, or otherwise amending the original list of objectives. Common sense dictates that the two parties change the list to reflect these newer situations. Common sense also suggests that in doing so they avoid the extreme of treating everything on the original list as worthless just because time has passed. The list is not cast in cement, nor is it to be torn into shreds ruthlessly: it is renegotiable.

Our recommended timeframe for the renewal of negotiations between superior and subordinate is quarterly. This is only because many MISs and other types of control systems are geared to quarterly reports. If your record-keeping or reporting system would fit a different timeframe, you should calendar your updates around what is most convenient and meaningful for you. The important thing here is that there be periodic updates and that both parties know in advance that there will be these *planned* opportunities for either to suggest a modification. That means they have to be scheduled, something the coordinator can remind people about. And it means objectives can be added, deleted or modified.

2. Problem-solving sessions. We learned in great detail in Chapter 11 how to get a group together for the purpose of brainstorming about a problem, defined as some result area in which performance is currently below par. Such unsatisfactory levels do not occur only when we are putting together a list of objectives. Performance could deteriorate any time during the year. Whenever we confront such a poor performance record, we should use the problem-solving approach to find appropriate solutions. Having these problem-solving sessions on a periodic basis is an excellent way of drawing attention to those result areas needing attention and updating the objectives list accordingly.

   In some hospitals the MBO coordinator monitors periodic reports and suggests a problem-solving session to the managers who identify unsatisfactory performance levels. In other institutions, the CEO will periodically dedicate time from routinely scheduled get-togethers (such as monthly department head meetings) to problem solving. What a good way to keep dynamic those meetings that all too often become a boring experience!

3. Innovative objectives. The list of objectives is supposed to include routine objectives, problem-solving objectives, and innovative objectives. Innovation does not wait until we are preparing objectives to introduce itself. Whenever in the course of the year a person comes up with a new idea of the sort we discussed in detail in Chapter 12, it should be written up and discussed as an innovative

objective. Those managers in particular who begin to be disenchanted with their own list of objectives as somehow preventing them from doing some of the things they would like to do should be invited to reduce what they'd like to do to innovative objectives and bring them in for negotiation. It could be that their earlier attempts to set objectives were a little divorced from the real world of their work and now that they've had a chance to think about what they want to do they have thought of some good ideas. Those ideas are usually not objectives, so such managers should be coached in the objective-writing skill and thereby given a chance to redo their list of objectives so it becomes vital and current in their eyes.

All managers should be alert to what are often called "targets of opportunity." These are objective areas that were not present when the list was originally negotiated but have surfaced since then as new opportunities to provide the service or otherwise fulfill the mission of the unit. Being able to include these in the list of objectives is a very important way of keeping the list current at all times, rather than waiting for next year or next quarter and run the risk of losing the opportunity to someone more "opportunistic."

4. VIP projects. Just as subordinates may wish to add new opportunities they see in the course of fulfilling their responsibilities, so the superior may at times come up with new projects, make new assignments. Rather than "dump" them on the subordinate in the shape of more work on top of an already busy schedule, both parties should discuss the new project as an innovative objective or as an additional KRA needing to be worked into some kind of an objective. Principles of good delegation tell the superior to define the results expected from such new work and not just assign the work. Because you can almost guarantee there will be some kind of VIP project for every one in the course of the year, a general rule to follow is to leave a little slack in the amount of time projected to achieve the original list of objectives when first negotiating them. Leave some slack that is to be taken up by these additional projects that will almost certainly arise sooner or later.
5. Longer-range objectives. Some objectives by their nature are projects that will take longer than one period of operation to accomplish. Some individuals, especially staff managers, may have an entire list of objectives made up of these longer-in-duration projects. In order that such a list of objectives be useful as any kind of a guide during the period of operations, it is especially important that attention be paid to identification of intermediate checkpoints so that some proximate objective (as one milestone along the way to the

completion of the project) always be kept in sight as a challenge. This is the only way such projects can be kept meaningful in the short run and can serve as reinforcement of success in the short run. Most often this is done by dividing the project into phases and selecting indicators of success for each phase. Such phases are analogous to making a first down on the football field. The goal line has not been crossed yet, so no points are scored, but as long as the team keeps making first downs (within a reasonable length of time), there is a sense of progress, heightened excitement, reward in keeping the ball, and further opportunities to get to the real objective.

WAYS TO FOLLOW UP

A third important series of techniques to help keep the system of MBO operational on a day-to-day basis after the original negotiating of objectives deals with ways to build in some follow-up procedures. Everyone needs a gentle reminder from time to time: some more than others. Here are a few ways you can build in follow-up:

1. Physical location of the objectives list. If the whole idea about objectives is that they are not to be written down only to be locked up in a file cabinet for 12 months and then be taken out to "see if we made them," then it follows that the list physically should not be filed away. If it is to serve as a daily reminder, perhaps it ought to be placed in a location where it can do exactly that: remind the managers of the commitment they made to each other and to the organization. What about placing them under the glass on the top of your desk? What about literally posting them on a bulletin board or some wall in the office? How about in a three-ring binder standing within reach on a shelf? You wouldn't lock your AAA road map, obtained to guide you in the family vacation, in a suitcase to be looked at once you arrived at your destination. So the guide for conducting the affairs of the work unit ought to be within ready reach for periodic examination and reference.
2. Establishing "present levels." In the negotiation process it sometimes happens that data are not readily available to insert in the "Present Level" column. In this case it was recommended that no commitment be made at the time with regard to future performance, since without knowledge of the present base of operations, no figure you pick for the future has much credibility. Instead it was suggested that in the columns labeled "Desired Level" be written the words

"Base to be established by ____(date)____." Whether you follow the precise method of documentation advised, or in some other way determine to begin tracking performance for that particular objective, you need to follow up on that later on. It would be the height of folly to return to the negotiation mode some months/years later and still find that you did not know what the present level of performance was. This means that the manager must set in motion some valid way of measuring the indicator in question and determine what the present performance level is and then follow up by negotiating a commitment for the period covered by the objectives at the next quarterly review session.

3. Tickler files. One of the functions of the coordinator of MBO in successful programs is to set up a master tickler file. This is any sort of follow-up reminder technique to serve as a stimulus to check that certain actions were performed or results obtained. Often it is 3″ × 5″ cards arranged chronologically by "suspense date" or due date. Or it could be notes made on a large enough calendar or in pocket calendars like the Day-Timer (trade name). The coordinator is doing this for the CEO to make note of the important events to be checked taken from all the objectives submitted in the master file.

   In like manner all managers might want to set up for themselves tickler files as a way to check progress on the acquisition of resources, on the completion of actions, on the attainment of completed objectives. These are all intermediate checkpoints along the way to successful completion of the year's work of the unit. Being reminded "automatically" by these files coming up for review like clockwork will help prevent forgetting about the objectives and will be a big aid in the allocation of the manager's time, thus staying out of the crisis-to-crisis syndrome.

SHOT-IN-THE-ARM EXAMPLES

All of the above techniques were mainly for the purpose of keeping the individual manager aware of the importance and usefulness of objectives in conducting business on a day-to-day basis. There is another group of procedures that is intended to give the entire MBO system a kind of shot-in-the-arm from time to time so that gradually, as happens in mature MBO programs, the word gets around that "here we manage by objectives as a way of life." Here are a few examples of how to do that:

1. Refresher courses. Most managers will have participated in some sort of introductory training session on the principles and practices

of MBO. The hospital's management development program ought to include refresher courses from time to time on the subject as a whole or on related subtopics such as personal development objectives, the art of negotiating, results-oriented performance appraisal, and the like. Whatever management education is provided ought to be results-oriented.

2. Readings on MBO. Some hospitals are able to support a management library that can be stocked with books on MBO and related topics. Any institution that formally implements MBO could at least purchase a few books on the topic aside from this one. Video tapes and other audiovisual aids are available for private or small group use on a selected basis. Sometimes the coordinator can work with the department of education in setting up review of such materials just prior to another round of negotiation sessions or performance reviews. Management journals and hospital literature occasionally print good articles on MBO that could be circulated among managers for their reading as a way of renewing interest and commitment to this way of managing the organization. You will find a list of recommended readings at the end of this book.
3. Evaluation of MBO. Implementing MBO was an innovative idea at one stage for your organization. Just as all innovations should be evaluated for their effectiveness in achieving desired results, so too MBO as a system should be evaluated to determine its success or failure. Chapter 19 describes the MBO usefulness survey, which we use for this purpose. Offshoots of doing such an evaluation are the renewed interest it brings on the part of managers and the opportunity it presents to recommit to MBO.
4. Hospital annual report. Somehow or other the CEO must make an annual report to the board of directors, to the stockholders, to the citizens, to the corporation, to the community at large. While this varies in formality from a closed session discussion in the conference room to a glossy-paper, multicolored printed annual report to a supplement in the local newspaper, there is always some kind of documentation serving as the official annual report. All managers ought to have special interest in this report because it records for posterity the accounting being made of how well the management team fulfilled its responsibility for conducting the affairs of the hospital. Hopefully many managers contributed to the report. At least all managers ought to be given a verbal report on its contents and a written copy of it. When this is done, the CEO can use this occasion as an authoritative opportunity to reinforce that MBO is "the way we manage this hospital" by couching his/her words in a way that

stresses what the objectives were and what the results were against those objectives.

SUMMARY

This chapter has stressed (1) the importance of keeping the objectives in mind—and physically in view—in order that they be the guide for day-to-day decision making that they were intended to be and (2) the consequent necessity of being sure that they are kept current and meaningful. Because the health care field is such a dynamic one with changes and improvements appearing constantly, it is impossible to look ahead in a list of objectives that covers one or more years and encompass every important result that the institution will need to achieve. *That is not the purpose of a list of objectives.* It is not supposed to be a forecast! It is a documentation of the meeting of the minds of two levels of management as to the currently understood contribution of each to the mission of the organization. If—or rather when—the need arises for a change in that agreement, the objectives should be modified to reflect the new understanding. Only in this way will both parties continue to feel safe in the belief that each knows what is on the other's mind.

Chapter 17

How to Evaluate by Objectives

In Chapter 7 we discounted the typical approach to performance appraisal as being more of a review of desirable personality traits that all too often turns out to be an opportunity for superiors to form subordinates into clones of themselves. This prevalent approach to performance review is so bad it is actually easy to make fun of it. But that would not be very productive unless we had something to offer in its stead. In MBO we do: It is called "results-oriented performance review."

Before studying the content of this chapter, it is important to remind yourself that all we discussed in the previous chapter relative to monitoring progress toward objectives was a type of evaluation. The managerial function of control is an ongoing one: you want to continuously evaluate actual performance against planned results. That is just part of the day-to-day job of managing. But every once in awhile, like maybe once a year, for the sake of good order you want to formalize that process a little and conduct what is often referred to as the *formal* performance evaluation of each of your people.

REASONS FOR FORMAL PERFORMANCE APPRAISAL

What we have in mind is another face-to-face meeting, another interview or two-way conversation. We might begin by asking why it might be a good idea to formalize this review process once a year through a formal interview between superior and subordinate.

Question: Why should you take the time once a year to sit down with each of your people individually to review performance?

Answer:

You probably mentioned several reasons for the formal performance interview. There are at least five major ones we think of. In checking your reasons against ours, pay special attention to the first and last, because that is where they belong, in our opinion, in terms of importance. We hold no special opinion on the priority of the others.

The first and primary reason for taking time on the job to formally review performance of an individual is *to try to improve performance on the job now held.* The most important reason for managers to devote time to this function is because it is one of their most effective ways of ensuring results on the job. In the course of the interview you will be controlling (checking *results* against plans); you will be organizing (adjusting resources to improve *results*); you will be directing (suggesting and ordering work activities to achieve *results*); you will be motivating (recognizing good *results,* encouraging even better *results*); you will be planning (identifying further desired *results*).

Notice the repeated use of the word *results:* this is results-oriented performance appraisal. The entire conversation during this interview is for the fundamental purpose of improving results on the job. This suggests that the appraisal procedure should not stop at an examination of the past; it should move on to the preparation of some plan for future action based on what has been learned in the past. If you discuss the activities and results of last year during the interview, it is not for the purpose of dangling skeletons from the closet in the face of your subordinates. If you have been managing at all throughout the year, they heard about unsatisfactory results when they happened. Instead, you look at them as though in a mirror, hoping they will reflect onto the future so performance in related areas can be bettered. Ask yourself, as a rough rule of thumb, about the last time you conducted a performance evaluation: *did you spend at least as much time talking about the future as you did talking about the past?* If you did not, you sold someone short. Personally, we think the whole process might be tremendously improved if only we started referring to it as the performance *pre*view!

A second basic purpose for the performance interview is the desire *to develop people.* Any manager should desire this because of two loyalties: (1) out of loyalty to the hospital you want to develop your people so there will be persons qualified to step into higher positions as they open up, and

(2) out of loyalty to your people you want to help them be ready for such a move when the occasion presents itself. One sure way of ruining morale and not developing pride in the kind of job done is to give the impression that your unit is a "dead-end" street, that all the new jobs are filled from outside the organization. Notice, then, that the discussion goes beyond the job now held and begins to consider potential future responsibilities, whether that means added duties in the present job position or promotion to a higher level position. You should be a help to the individual who wishes to acquire the knowledge, skills, and/or attitudes needed for those new responsibilities. Here then is the perfect time to discuss personal development objectives along the lines discussed in detail in Chapter 13. Ask yourself again, about the last time you conducted a performance evaluation: *did you spend time talking about the personal development needs of your people?*

A third basic reason for the performance review (almost inseparable from the previous one), is to provide answers to the two questions that seem to be the recurrent concern of almost every organization member: *"How am I doing?"* and *"Where do I go from here?"* Answers are of obvious benefit to the people whose minds they occupy. They can also be of great value to the hospital because in many cases these questions so preoccupy individuals that they prevent them from hearing or responding to anything else.

It is only human for an individual to want these questions answered from time to time. The child seeks recognition from the parents: "Look at me, Mommy; tell me what a good boy (girl) I am." The student needs recognition from the teacher, so we have tests and grades and honors. The employees, even professionals, need reassurance from the organization that their contribution is recognized, is meaningful, is deserving of reward. It is you as the management representative of the hospital who is called upon to answer these questions for each of your people.

Our observation of executives completing performance appraisals indicates that only some 50% of them give direct answers to those questions.

Question: Why is it that some 50% of managers shy away from leveling with their subordinates about the precise worth of their performance?

Answer:

You could have cited any one of a number of reasons. The first would be that in many cases the superior probably had no measurable way of determining satisfactory performance. It is very hard to tell individuals precisely how well they are performing if you have never figured out with them how to measure performance. Objectives will remedy this.

Besides that, we found the most common reasons for lack of honest evaluations are the many facets of the superior's insecurity. If you are insecure yourself, you will tend not to make forthright evaluations because of fear. If you are dealing with excellent performers, you will tend to be less than honest with them because an excellent rating will bring a request for rewards, and you might not be able to deliver any. Or an excellent rating could give subordinates ideas about promotion and you do not want to lose them, so you discount some successes. Or an excellent rating could make a person think about wanting your job. Now you are really fearful, so once again you avoid that by simply not being candid.

If you're dealing with a marginal performer, you might also tend to be less than honest because that's hard work. If you have to find fault, you had better be able to substantiate it. That means work, and it might even mean you are in danger of being accused of judging someone else's "professionalism." That's always risky, so insecurity wins out. Or if you are willing to bite the bullet and confront subordinates with hard evidence, they may sulk because you do not know how to say it right. That only means more work motivating again, so the easy way out is to forget it. Or in the worst case, an honest review might cause the person to actually quit, and you sure do not want that to happen because then you would be short-handed, or you might get an even less capable replacement, so once again you take the easy way out.

You want to anticipate those questions and bring them up even if the subordinate never gets around to verbalizing them: "How am I doing?" "Where might I go from here?" and "What are we going to do to get me ready for that?" which is the logical follow-up on considering the future. Ask yourself, the last time you conducted a performance review, *did you give direct answers to these questions that all subordinates want answered?* If not, you sold somebody short.

A fourth reason for taking the time to conduct a good performance review is to provide a basis for coordinating the hospital, department, and individual objectives. From a motivational point of view, as well as from a results point of view, it is important from time to time to cement the interrelationship of objectives at all levels of the institution. You want to take this opportunity, periodically then, of blending the individual's objectives into those of the organization.

When discussing the successes, you want to impress upon subordinates that they were the basis for your own success and for the success of the hospital, that one is directly tied to the other. When discussing failures, you also want to point out the domino effect they have had: their failures meant you failed in part in the entire work unit, and that, in all probability, meant a degree of failure in one of the hospital's objectives. This is the way to build teamwork. We sink or swim together. The last time you conducted a performance review, *did you take the opportunity to build team spirit?* If you didn't, you sold everyone short.

A fifth and least important reason, in our judgment, for performance review is to provide necessary documentation for appropriate personnel actions. This aspect of the review has been overstressed in the past and has been the basis for much of the opposition to evaluations. While it is true that in a complex organization we need documentation of performance records, appraisals, and recommendations, the documentation is only the tail and should not wag the dog.

You don't want to invite your people to sit down and go over the performance evaluation form so "we can send it to Personnel." This is putting the cart before the horse. Rather, you should invite them to sit down and discuss the other points listed here, and only as a matter of good record keeping advise other offices of the judgments you jointly are making about the individual's present and future contribution to the hospital.

In examining your own record on this point in the past, check also which individuals seem to receive less than reasonable amounts of your time. If you are failing in this fifth dimension of performance appraisal, you may find yourself saying to the better workers "I know there's only a couple minutes left before we both have to dash home, but come in here for a couple of seconds and sign this review form, will you, so that we can satisfy Personnel and get you your salary adjustment?" The inference is that individuals who are good performers do not need much of your time in this very important aspect of your managerial relationship; only the "problem children" or "troublemakers" get a large chunk of your time. How short-sighted! Your better people need *strokes* as well as your poorer ones. As a matter of fact, your better people are your major assets, and if you don't spend time building on your strong people, your organization will not be maximizing its resources.

STEP-BY-STEP PROCEDURE

If these five purposes of the appraisal interview are to be accomplished, there should be a step-by-step procedure instituted to ensure the right kind of evaluations. Following the pattern of mutual objective-setting discussed in earlier chapters, we recommend the following similar sequence of events.

Employee Self-Appraisal

Just prior to the scheduled time for an appraisal interview, individuals should prepare a memorandum to their superior summarizing evaluations of themselves. The memorandum should include:

- the objectives agreed upon at the beginning of the year
- the results achieved for each objective
- any extenuating circumstances involved where objectives were not met
- any accomplishments that go beyond the previously agreed-upon objectives
- a list of areas for personal growth as seen by the individual for his/her own improvement on the job and by way of preparation for future assignments in his/her career

Supervisor Tentative Evaluation

At about the same time, you should make an independent summary judgment about the past performance of the individual. You could have a preprinted form designed for this purpose. It is hoped that it will not stress personality traits. Rather, it should cover:

- accomplished results compared with desired results
- extenuating circumstances to explain objectives not met
- additional accomplishments beyond agreed-upon objectives
- personal development needs you would like to point out to the individual for present or future assignments (knowledge, skills, attitudes)
- summary judgment about the overall worth of the individual to the hospital

One-on-One Interview

In this interview you want to compare notes with the individual about performance and future potential. The following points are offered as a general guide only to assist in conducting the discussion. (Detailed courses in interviewing, coaching, and counseling are available for this purpose.)

1. Establish a friendly atmosphere by selecting the right time and place for the interview. Be sure the interview will be free from interruptions.

2. Plan the interview carefully, selecting two or three key points that you want to be sure to get across before the discussion is over. Do not make the interview sound as though these are the only things on your mind, however.
3. Let the employee talk first, discussing the summary memo prepared. Be alert to this discussion for opportunities that might help you inject the two or three main points you have on your mind.
4. Concentrate on the positive aspects of performance and offer constructive criticism pointing the way to future development. Rehashing past errors and failures should be done only to illustrate possible development needs. Remember you should have had quarterly opportunities to discuss these points, so make this year-end summary exactly that, a summary rather than a rehash.
5. Encourage the individual to analyze his/her own performance to determine areas of weakness and areas of strength. Ask questions such as "What do you believe may have caused that project to fail/succeed?"
6. At times you might have to take the initiative, and as a coach or counselor, point out why performance failed or succeeded, what strengths and weaknesses are, how improvement might be achieved in the future.
7. Make certain the discussion stays on specifics, on measurable results. Do not get bogged down in arguments about minutiae.
8. Be sure to cover priorities so sufficient groundwork has been laid for preparing a list of objectives for the next operational period.
9. Get a commitment as to work to be done to satisfy personal development needs.
10. Be willing to modify your preliminary judgments about performance based on new information and insights brought to your attention by the individual. This is why your earlier judgment was considered tentative. Try not to lead the discussion as a way to prove your early judgment was correct: you win, the other party loses!
11. Make a final overall judgment about the individual, progress to date, worth to the hospital, as well as any recommendations (of a personal nature) you might be expected to make on the written instrument. Share all this with the individual. Be sure he/she understands your judgment, even if not agreeing with it. Get a signature and explain that the signature does not necessarily signify the person agrees with your judgment, but does understand it. Avoid in this summary judgment falling prey to the "halo effect" (thinking the individual is a saint because of one good recent result) or the

"horns effect" (thinking the individual is a devil because of one bad recent result).

Follow-up during the Year

Set up and maintain a performance file on each individual during the course of the year. To assist in making a meaningful appraisal the next time around, you should keep a record of memos, reports, revised objectives, and the like that occur during the year and would be useful in the results-oriented performance review. For example, you might take note of:

- successful completion of an objective (or stage of one)
- initiation or completion of a phase of a personal development objective
- notice of an unforeseen problem encountered that could affect the completion of performance or development objectives
- notice of developing conditions or factors that could affect performance activities (new equipment, organizational changes, etc.)
- periodic budget and expense reports
- outstanding or unusual achievements in performance
- constructive criticisms or disciplinary interviews
- coaching or counseling interviews
- revision of objectives
- complaints received about the person and his/her work
- commendations received because of the person and/or the person's work
- notes made during quarterly reviews with the individual

Personal Development Needs

The reader will have noted that in much of this discussion we made constant reference to personal development. It is hoped that the people you are coaching received the impression that one of your primary concerns during performance review is their personal growth. Whenever areas of unsatisfactory performance are being discussed and you probe for contributing causes, you might have occasion to mention the person's failings. Maybe it is some information/knowledge that is missing. Maybe it is due to an attitude (lack of appreciation, lack of incentive, immaturity, or prejudice of one sort or another). Maybe it is due to lack of some skill.

Be sure to spend time during the review to help the individual identify these to lay the groundwork for personal development objectives.

A Final Word about Forms

Whenever performance review is the topic of discussion, the most common request is, "Do you have a sample evaluation form that is a good one that we can use?" We have tried to resist the temptation to offer a model form in response to this anticipated question, not because we have never seen a good one, rather, because most people simply take someone else's and copy it instead of using it as a basis for design of one to meet individual local needs.

The critical point is that whatever form you design to meet documentation requirements be results-oriented. The list of points to be covered that we set forth above emphasized results. If you get those points in somehow, you will have a satisfactory form. By way of frosting on the cake, you may want to weight the objectives, so you will have a weighting column. You may want to base a bonus program on results, so you will mathematically compute a bonus by establishing bonus points for each objective. You may want to explore personality and attitudinal characteristics as background for present performance and future considerations, so you will add a section with room for those judgments. There is no one form to meet your needs, so design your own.

SUMMARY

Self-appraisal is a vital part of participative management. When individuals share the burden of their appraisal with their superior, they approach the performance review situation with a significantly different attitude. When invited, urged, and assisted by the procedure to appraise their own performance, appraisal is colored by the knowledge that they play a vital role in shaping their own destiny. In actuality, each person should assume such a role as a participating member of the management team. The feelings of futility, frustration, and antagonism toward the superior and "management" typically experienced in appraisal systems in which individuals are called in, allowed to read a completed review, and informed of their status—no questions asked or tolerated—are not apt to exist under the philosophy of self-appraisal.

Another aspect of self-appraisal has been recognized in this chapter. We grow and learn through experience on the job. It is easy, however, to become so involved with the day-to-day process of managing or getting our work done that we have little time or inclination to really study and analyze what we have been doing. The self-appraisal element of the performance review forces us to study, analyze, and give critical attention to self and to where we are and where we want to go. We gain new insights and we continue to grow.

There is no such thing as an easy performance review. It continues to be one of the most difficult responsibilities of all managers. It is, however, one of the most fundamental and potentially the most productive of all the manager's many duties. When the concept of growth and development of the individual becomes the central concern of the performance review, the door is opened in a nonthreatening way for periodic discussion of growth potential. Only then can we begin to gain confidence as managers that we are actively working to actuate all possible potential in ourselves as well as our subordinates.

Chapter 18

Implementation Strategies

We have now examined each of the steps outlined in Chapter 3 for a complete system of MBO, and we have practiced writing each of the kinds of objectives in a complete system of MBO. We have also seen how to record progress along the way and how to conduct a formal results-oriented performance review.

You have, in a word, seen all the pieces of the system and should be ready to implement. It is now *your* turn to ask a few questions that might be on your mind at this time. This chapter records some commonly asked questions dealing with strategies of implementation and offers some thoughts (as opposed to hard and fast answers) you might like to consider in mapping your strategies.

Question: How do you get the doctors to cooperate?

Hospital-based physicians have always been a challenge to MBO. For many years CEOs have had to work very carefully with chiefs of radiology and chiefs of laboratory, in particular, in order to secure cooperation in MBO. In recent years new physician executives have been added in many hospitals, such as chiefs of medicine, surgery, and pediatrics, that are even a greater challenge in installing MBO. Nevertheless, they can be made a part of the MBO team. It is up to the CEO to achieve this relationship. The CEO should start by having the MBO program formally approved by the board of trustees. In addition, discussion at and approval by the joint conference committee would be useful. Thereupon it can be brought up for information at the medical staff executive committee. The strategy here is to be firm, consistent, and helpful. Don't try to rush it but keep a steady course. It can be done.

Question: How long does it take to implement such a full-blown system of MBO?

The literature, based on experiences of organizations to date, suggests a three- to five-year timeframe. This does not mean it will take that long to teach and inaugurate the system. It means that, given the long time to complete the cycle of plan → work → review (i.e., a 12-month period to complete the cycle), and since most people need to repeat anything a few times before they become proficient in it, it follows that it will be three to five year-long cycles before most managers will feel comfortable with it as a way of life.

Question: But how long will it take to get various levels of managers in our hospital actually working under an objectives system?

If a formal commitment is made, starting with the CEO and executive committee, and if the sequence of events is scheduled as recommended in Chapter 3, a three-month period of concentrated effort can launch the system very effectively. The first month would be spent by the administration in reviewing the mission statement, updating the long-range plan, doing a needs analysis, and writing the hospitalwide objectives. The second month would be used for training of department heads, preparation of their departmental goals, and negotiating their goals with administration. The third month would repeat the same for supervisors within each department.

Question: What assumptions does this kind of timetable make regarding resources to bring it off smoothly?

Again, assuming commitment from the top and the courage to require cooperation in meeting schedules, the only other resource needed would be an internal coordinator of MBO. (The job description for this individual was given in Chapter 3.) This person might use an outside consultant for certain key functions, such as conducting the training sessions, facilitating the group needs analysis and objective-setting discussions, or tutoring individuals in their first list of objectives. If such help is used, the coordinator should be present at all meetings to learn from the consultant and not rely any longer than necessary on such an outside crutch. Minimal expenses will be involved in other aids such as training materials (e.g., extra copies of this volume), internally devised forms, and the like.

Question: How do you know whom to appoint as MBO coordinator?

This is a staff appointment and therefore requires the ability to serve as an adviser to offer advice, to see that necessary controls are set up. Not everyone can handle this. You would not want to select someone with no influence at all on others, for there will be times when a little good-natured arm-twisting will be called for. You would not want to select someone who would try to give orders to people about their role in MBO, for this would invite discontent not only with the coordinator, but with the whole idea of objectives. You would not want it to be the CEO, because it is a time-consuming job at the outset (up to half time for the three-month introductory period) and because the CEO also needs the kind of good-natured prodding called for to keep the system on a time schedule.

You might want to select someone close to the top (an assistant administrator, an administrative resident, a key division head). Try to keep it out of personnel or training because then it tends to be seen as "another training program."

Question: Is it necessary to commit the entire hospital to this system from the outset?

You will recall a brief discussion at the beginning of Chapter 3 about the wisdom of total implementation versus a modular approach. While this volume has recommended total immersion, there is also the possible strategy of implementing more gradually.

After all, implementing MBO is an innovative idea, and we saw in our discussion of innovations in Chapter 12 that a pilot project is often a beginning step. You might wish to set objectives only at the administrative level first, or only down through department heads, and only if it proves worthwhile to go further down in the organization.

Or, you could take a vertical slice of the organization: that is, implement first only in fiscal affairs, or in nursing service, or some other group of departments—but involving all levels of management. Then, if the pilot proves worthwhile, other departments will be anxious to do the same.

Question: If we choose the piecemeal approach, how do we know which areas to involve first?

This is another important strategy. Some will choose to work first with those managers who seem to be most anxious, most supportive, most interested in making it work. Others will choose those areas where it is easier to measure results, such as the business office or clinical departments with readily identifiable work units like radiology or the laboratory.

Somewhat more questionable is the strategy employed by others who deliberately choose as the trial unit the one whose manager is a cynic. The reasoning seems to be, "So-and-so is our tough nut, and if we don't get support there, this system will never work, so let's find out from the start if we're going to be accepted there!''

Question: Wherever we start, how will we know if the system is worthwhile?

Again, if MBO is an innovation, it must produce certain benefits to offset the associated costs of time and energy, or it must be considered a failure. In the first chapter we suggested that some of the more general advantages to any management team are improved planning, improved motivation, and improved communication. But these are themselves only means to the more definite end of improved performance.

You could do a prestudy and poststudy by checking the current level of planning, motivation, and communications in the hospital before the start of MBO and again after it has been in use for a year or two. Many hospitals do periodic attitude surveys of supervisors and employees. Several questions in those surveys could be selected (or added) as yardsticks for measuring change. MBO will not be the only variable contributing to any change but usually can be identified as to its degree of influence on the change.

More specifically, you should have a definite objective or two in mind for introducing MBO. The very purpose of MBO is to help people clarify in their mind what they intend to accomplish by various work programs. Then, shouldn't you do the same thing with MBO? Clarify before you implement precisely what you hope to achieve. Perhaps you desire greater incidence of department heads jointly planning their work; or maybe you seek more decisions being made at a lower level in the organization; or it could be your primary aim is a hospital-wide attack on certain common problems such as late charges, turnover, cost control, or some clinical deficiency. Any or all these could then be used as a way of checking the success of the system of MBO.

Question: How many objectives should there be?

There are no hard and fast rules about this. The intent of a person's list of objectives is to record measurable results for all of his/her major areas of responsibilities. The word ''major'' means right away that the list is selective and limited to the big items. Therefore, having a hundred objectives is too many! But most managers will have more than one or two major responsibilities, so one or two objectives is probably not enough!

It was suggested that the CEO might have fifteen to twenty objectives, while department heads might have ten to fifteen each, and supervisors eight to ten each. The number is higher at a higher level to show a broader scope of responsibility at the top and to recognize that first-level supervisors are, in part, working supervisors. Since objectives at any level are the personal objectives of the manager at that level, there cannot be many more than this at any level, however, or the list will be unrealistic.

It is usually the case that supervisors will have less experience/sophistication in measuring their results, and this is an added reason to suggest fewer at that level. A good maxim here might be: better to have a few meaningful, well-done objectives than a lot of poor ones.

Question: You keep mentioning annual objectives. Is that the only time frame used?

What a manager can accomplish by way of results is normally dependent on available resources. (Not that money and people should dictate objectives, because the preferable sequence is to decide the results you want, then figure out the work to get those results, and then obtain resources to do that work!) But resources are normally allocated on some sort of a budgetary cycle, typically twelve months (or thirteen four-week periods in some organizations). It makes sense then to have the time you covered by objectives coincide with the time span covered by the budget. And many institutions now begin considering next year's objectives when they start putting together next year's budget. This is usually an up-down-up process covering several months of the calendar; so should be the iterative objective-setting process.

As an alternative strategy for the first go-around, which is often a learning process, you might consider a six-month or so time frame. This way you can pay attention to starting the system well without at the same time worrying about budget meetings and the like—anything to minimize diversions during the training and start-up time! A shorter first-time through often helps reduce fear of the system and provides a more relaxed atmosphere to learn it.

Question: Are there other caveats about timing the initial implementation?

You might reflect for awhile on the points raised in Chapter 2 about the managerial climate. There the emphasis was on participation and openness to allow for proper negotiating of desired results.

Akin to that is anything else that might militate against calm, deliberate, and trustful negotiating. If, for example, there has just been a change in the top management (a new CEO, a merger, an acquisition), that would probably not be an appropriate time to inaugurate MBO. New relationships of mutual respect and trust should be established first.

Or, if your hospital is in the middle of moving to a new building or expanding considerably in bed size, this would probably not be an appropriate time to start MBO. The management team is doubtless experiencing enough trauma without the additional unsettling of having to learn to set objectives. (If MBO could be installed prior to the move or expansion, it might be a big help in an orderly transition.)

Question: How far "down the ranks," so to speak, do you go in setting objectives?

This system is typically called a way of managing managers. That is to say it is usually used down as far as the first-level supervisor, who negotiates with his/her superior. There is a historical reason for this. Measuring managers by their results is a Johnny-come-lately. We say that the formal system of MBO goes back to Peter Drucker's first book, *The Practice of Management,* published in 1954, which described management practices for a short time prior to the publication date. But others in the work force had been measured in their performance long before that. Production people have been measured since the days of scientific management and the industrial engineers (turn of the century). Union workers have been measured by contract provisions since the mid-1800s. Office workers have had "work measurement" programs since the 1920s.

During all that time there was no concerted effort to measure the contribution of managers to the results of the organization. MBO fills that unmet need. It doesn't seem wise to go back now and superimpose this new system on top of previously existing ones (unless they are not doing the job).

Question: What about people who aren't supervisors but who don't fall into the categories you just mentioned?

In a hospital there will be many such persons: they do not have a supervisor's title and do not, therefore, manage people, but they are not hourly employees. This will include many salaried professionals and paraprofessionals such as nurses, technicians, administrative assistants, analysts, researchers, instructors, counselors. If they manage resources of the hospital other than people (time, money, equipment) and if they have some discretion about making decisions or using these resources, then you might very well wish to involve them in negotiating objectives.

Discretion is the key word. Production workers, union employees, and office workers under time and motion studies do not have much discretion, so they cannot very well negotiate. But where discretion exists, there ought to be accountability for those decisions.

Question: How do we record our agreed-upon objectives?

In the course of practicing our objectives for this book, we used several different formats for recording our thoughts. These several formats were for the purpose of being sure the parties negotiating the goals arrived at a complete meeting of the minds about the real commitment intended by the objective. For routine objectives, it was a commitment to meet certain standards; for problem-solving objectives, it was a commitment to solve the problems; for innovative objectives, it was a commitment to added benefits; for personal development objectives, it was a commitment to individual effort dealing with knowledge, skills, or attitudes.

But once information is all agreed upon, the summary of the commitment can be reduced to a single form, which accommodates all types.

All you need to design a suitable form is to begin with the columns we worked with for the routine objectives (Exhibit 10-1). Add a final column headed "Program," and you have all you need to include additional pertinent information for problem-solving, innovative, and personal development goals.

Question: How important is it to tie in the appraisal or money aspect to objectives?

It was suggested in Chapter 7 that appraisal is the logical conclusion of the system. It comes last in the sequence of steps and last in importance as a reason for implementing. To do otherwise invites misinterpretation as to why objectives are set at all. There are always those who are convinced that administration is simply looking for a way to chop heads.

Now that's a lot different from saying you can do without any appraisal or rewards based on performance. Time and again systems have been implemented with no teeth in them, and performance has not changed one bit. The logic of the system requires that commitments be rewarded/punished in accord with performance. If it is fair for superiors not to use objectives as a hatchet, it is also fair for subordinates to accept the consequences of their actions.

A strategy sometimes used is to defer the monetary correction until participants in the system have had a couple of passes at setting objectives and have acquired the knack of it. Then there will be less fear and less of a tendency to "pad" the objectives to get a raise by looking good.

Another strategy, always to be encouraged, is to separate the discussion of money rewards from the discussion of performance. There can be a *logical* connection between these two topics but a chronological separation in the conversations. This means during the performance review session, the subordinate is made to understand performance is the basis for decisions about raises, but the actual discussion of how much will be left to a later date. (Many organizations try to even out the impact of salary adjustments in their cash flow by spreading the raises over the year and having only a percentage take effect each quarter or each month.)

Question: What is the worst mistake we can make in seeking to implement MBO?

Despite all the positive and promising comments made about MBO in this book, the worst mistake would be to be guilty of oversell. This can be seen in the several kinds of behavior, such as announcing and treating MBO as a panacea. It might be the best system of management known to date, but it will not cure all your ills because it is a people-oriented system and will require people to make it work. Also to be discouraged is suggesting that what managers did before was imperfect, amateurish, unsophisticated, or otherwise bad, whereas now MBO is going to get them to behave entirely differently. The exact opposite would be a much more desirable strategy: suggesting managers have already been doing a lot of what we call MBO, and now you are simply trying to formalize it all and make it uniform.

Running a quick "training" session and thinking everyone will be so enamored with the self-evident advantages of MBO as to become overnight wizards at setting objectives is another pitfall. Not everyone will react with the same degree of acceptance, so not everyone will even try hard at once. With all, a planned sequence of experiences will be more helpful to gradually awaken interest and desire. Above all, do not get upset with uneven abilities in setting objectives, measuring results, and so forth. Your managers have varying skills, varying interests, and you will have to be patient with varying results in using the system.

In a word, be patient with yourself and with others. . . .

Question: When setting departmental objectives, what are some good criteria to use in determining which objectives should be written for the department?

It might be useful to consider the head of the department as a kind of CEO who will want to set objectives much as the CEO of the hospital does. That is, to be used for two purposes: first, to see whether managers are adequately discharging all the responsibilities entrusted to them in being put in charge, and second, as a cue that others in the department are to take their lead in knowing what is expected of them. Hence, the selection of objectives should be done in a way that these two purposes are able to be fulfilled. Let the department head ask: (1) Which areas do I know I am accountable to administration for in running this department? (That includes accountabilities horizontally to other departments and service units.) (2) What areas do I wish to call to the attention of others within the department so that they will know they are high in priority and thus to be reflecting on their individual lists of objectives?

Question: What questions should I ask when trying to narrow an objective statement to only those areas for which I have control?

The critical word in accepting accountability is not the word *control.* There are few duties we have in which we are able to control the many variables that will affect the outcome, if we take control in the literal sense. But we are responsible for many areas that we are expected to be able to *influence.* The difference of course is in the way in which we have an impact. When you control something, you can order it to occur; you can order the circumstances that will make it occur; you can direct the activities of those who will make it happen. When you influence something, you use persuasion rather than orders; you use motivation rather than direction; you sell an idea rather than telling it. So the questions to ask might better be couched in terms of your ability to influence. "Is there any way in which I might be expected to influence the outcome?" "Are there any circumstances that I can influence to change?" "Will I be in a position to influence the other individuals involved in bringing about the result?" "Do I have enough influence in the particular area to make a difference in the way it turns out?"

Question: Can a hospital unit have an effective MBO program without a corporate commitment and participation in the program?

Earlier in the text we used the analogy of a pie, suggesting that half a pie might be better than no pie at all. Ideally implemented, MBO must start at the corporate level and eventually involve all units. But sometimes we have to settle for less than the ideal and can do so with less than ideal effectiveness. There is a readily understandable correlation between the degree of effectiveness and the degree of autonomy of the hospital unit in question. The more autonomy, the less harm is done by lack of corporate support and involvement. Thus a free standing and geographically separate hospital unit (one hospital in a group, a separate ambulatory care unit, a free-standing surgicenter, a satellite operation) will be able to have an effective program within the confines of its own four walls, especially if it has control of its own budget and is treated as a separate profit center. Even within a given hospital, a single operating department can have an effective program as long as there is a lot of autonomy in the conduct of daily operations; for example, an outpatient services unit with its own medical records, radiology, and lab support.

Question: How can we help those who get hung up on their particular objectives not being what they really do most of the time?

This is the person who probably for the first time has been forced to think in terms of results at the end of a day or a series of days, rather than looking at one activity after another. If the objectives list really does state the results of the individual's work responsibilities, it is related to the person's daily work but is not a list of events. Try to get such individuals to see beyond "what they do most of the day" to why those things are done, to the desired results that cause them to be done.

Question: What is the role of the outside consultant in establishing a system of MBO?

Management theorists and practitioners have agreed that no one else can manage for you, that you cannot delegate your managerial responsibilities to someone else. You may get help from others inside and outside the organization in the fulfilling of this or that function of management, but they remain helpers while you remain the manager.

We deliberately begin our answer on the role of a consultant as a change agent in establishing a system of MBO with this caveat because it tells us clearly what the consultant's role is *not*. It is not to make decisions: the manager does that. It is not to implement any system of management: the manager does that. It is not to replace the manager in whole or in part, but to assist.

There are countless studies we could share with you in which the implementation of MBO just plain failed. Most of those are instances in which CEOs expected or allowed internal or external consultants to "get this damn program going" either because it was the thing to do these days or because some agency or board of trustees or governmental body mandated the implementation. Management will always be a highly personal responsibility, one that must involve the presence and the active involvement of the person who is the manager. And any system of management that does not start with this premise is doomed to failure.

What *is* the role of the consultant then? We have found a threefold role to be appropriate: (1) the consultant gives advice; (2) the consultant is a teacher or trainer; (3) the consultant is a facilitator.

The Consultant as Adviser. We don't happen to like the word *expert,* but you go to consultants first of all because they are felt to know a little more about a topic than you do. Consultants have specialized in a particular field because they have more time to devote to that area than you do, given your many other responsibilities. Consultants are eclectics: they bring to you the breadth of experiences they have had with a variety of organizations, some similar and some not so similar, and you expect them to draw from these experiences to give advice on your situation.

When it comes to MBO, because of the personal characteristic of the management position, you will seek this kind of help from the consultants; that is, based on their experience elsewhere, you will want advice on such matters as:

- Should we even get into MBO?
- Are we ready for it yet, or are there some preliminaries we should get taken care of first?
- What is the proper timing for starting such a system?
- What strategies are there to select from in implementing?
- Where do we start?
- Can it work in a part of the organization?
- What are the steps normally followed?
- What are the pitfalls to watch out for?
- What resources should be committed to the system?

In a word, you go to consultants to tailor make the implementation of such a system to fit you as manager and your organization.

The Consultant as Trainer. Orientation and training sessions are very much needed early on in the implementation of MBO. An understanding of the principles and a certain amount of skill in the procedures of MBO must be achieved by many individuals. Assuming that individuals know how to manage or that they can simply be told to start negotiating objectives is exactly what has been done in the past and why many organizations now realize the need for formally implementing MBO. If you as the manager attempt to provide this training for your people, you will be slighting other duties, and you may candidly be perceived as a manipulator of some sort, trying to "pull" something on those of your administrators and staff who need most to have their thinking reoriented.

Many with positions of authority in your institution believe:

> We are different here. This is a hospital. We deal with people, with health, with intangibles. This is not a business where you manufacture and sell material things to make a profit. Those methods won't fit us; people from General Motors have nothing to offer us.

Up until the last clause there is no argument. Hospitals are different, hospitals deal with people, with health, with intangibles. The objective is not increased production, increased sales, or increased profits (necessarily). All true. But before one can correctly conclude that the methods of General Motors or other business managers cannot be helpful, one must first demonstrate that they do not also deal with people, with intangibles, with the physical, emotional, and ecological well-being of people as well as with tangible products. The effort of MBO then is not to turn hospital managers into GM executives. It is to learn to apply some of the techniques of the modern professional manager who is at home in a business firm, a unit of government, a hospital, the Boy Scouts of America, a major university.

Physicians in particular are prone to prejudge MBO, either because of a bad experience they saw or heard about, or because of a simple lack of sufficient study of what it's all about. The fear they have is that MBO will impose structure, hierarchy, and narrowly directed behavior on an organization and a profession that they believe is supposed to be free, open, and dedicated to their trained judgment.

Consultants are often able to point out that such fears are baseless. All purposeful organizations are faced with the need to agree on objectives to which the group will orient, to choose from alternative strategies to reach the established objectives, to reduce the selected strategy to achievable tasks, to establish a timeframe within which progress toward the objectives will be measured, and to marshall/allocate/coordinate the flow of human, material, information, and energy resources to effect the program.

If the hospital CEO says something like that, staff often hear it as the expected party line, and no change takes place. Consultants can and do get into dialogue with staff about such a simple statement and often succeed in getting behavioral and attitudinal change.

Other simply erroneous impressions about MBO, especially on the part of professionals, can be dealt with in similar fashion. They can be helped to see that MBO is not what they presumed based on rumor. Usually the consultant has run into these attitudes before and once again draws on experience to aid in effecting change.

The Consultant as Facilitator. Once plans are made to fit the needs of the particular hospital, once training sessions are carried out to enhance understanding and ability to plan and evaluate health care objectives, the promise of a successful MBO implementation becomes great. But it will then depend on the ability of the key administrators to bring it off according to promise. In particular it becomes the challenge of the CEO to start the process. Not to order the process, but to start it.

Some senior executives believe in the system but doubt their own ability to lead the process. And well they might: often they are not personally trained any more than their colleagues in doing a needs analysis, in formulating measurable objectives, in negotiating supportive objectives, in monitoring progress, in following up on the details of documentation. Any and all of these task elements are among the areas in which consultants come in next. They typically are trained as facilitators in group process techniques, in various styles of management, in negotiating procedures, in forms design and data collection. But in all of these areas it should be remembered again that the consultant is a helper; you must still manage. The consultant cannot negotiate objectives for you, or determine the educational or other needs of your patients, or set priorities for you, or arbitrate the differences of opinion among your staff. Assist—yes; facilitate—yes; do it for or without you—no!

A good consultant will try to become expendable as time goes by. After you lean on this crutch for awhile, you learn to throw away the crutch. You will need someone in a staff capacity to keep the details flowing. This is your MBO coordinator, about which much has been said in Chapter 3. This individual will have worked closely with the outside consultant, getting ready to assume those responsibilities as well as the ones set out in the coordinator's job description.

SUMMARY

This chapter has reviewed some of the more common questions asked by those beginning to implement MBO in the formal sense outlined in this book, as well as by those who wish to review their progress some time later.

Chapter 19

How to Evaluate the Success of Your Implementation of MBO

Much has been said and written, here and elsewhere, about the potential usefulness of MBO as a system of management for health care institutions and other organizations. You may be one of those health care managers who has implemented one form or another of MBO in the hope of realizing some of its touted benefits. You will then wish to evaluate whether the system is working or not.

The typical discussion about the effectiveness of MBO in the literature tends to be a list of the more common inadequacies of most attempts to implement.[1] Among the difficulties thus identified are failings such as:

- lack of awareness of the rationale or value of MBO on the part of many managers
- insufficient real negotiations in the setting of objectives
- insufficient time spent reviewing progress during the course of the year
- a feeling that the system is too formal or too rigid
- inadequate knowledge in the organization about top management's real objectives and priorities
- lack of understanding of how to negotiate, how to measure, how to follow up
- need for more patience, flexibility, and practice

The purpose of this chapter is to suggest a more objective method of evaluation of the success or failure of your implementation of MBO. It is based on the same premise advanced in our earlier discussion of innovative objectives. Implementation of something new is not a success unless it achieves the added benefits for the organization that were the determining factors leading to the decision to implement. Our contention all along has been that MBO is adopted as a means to do a better job in achieving the mission of the organization. Therefore MBO is a success only to the degree that it helps carry out the mission, which is measured by achievement of agreed-upon objectives. Since every hospital has its unique mission and objectives, your MBO system will be a success to the degree that you succeed in achieving your objectives. The same would be true about any system of management.

We also made the claim in Chapter 1 that MBO does all this because it helps managers perform their specific functions, their contribution to the achievement of objectives. In particular, its procedures are geared at:

1. improved planning
2. improved communicating
3. improved motivation

In general, MBO is to help managers do their job by helping them "to stay on the front wheel of the bicycle," to keep the organization going towards desired results, rather than just getting lost in all the activities represented by the flurry of the back wheel of the bicycle.

It would seem that a fair way to evaluate the success in implementing such a system would be to ask the managers using the system if they find it helpful in the carrying out of these managerial responsibilities. With the assistance of the CEO and MBO coordinator of each hospital, we surveyed managers of 24 hospitals using the approach to MBO described in this book.[2] In some instances we followed up with verbal interviews. The heart of the survey was a 53-item questionnaire, answered anonymously. Room for freely offered additional comments was also provided. Five additional questions about the respondents' background were asked, so that for each item of satisfaction the responses could be tabulated and analyzed based on a person's training in MBO, level in the organization, length of time as a manager, work area, and years of experience with MBO.

For each question in the survey, five choices were available to the respondent, on a scale of 1 to 5, usually going from *strongly agree* to *strongly disagree* with the statement. The mean response value for each was computed and reported to each hospital. The mean response value on the same item as answered by all other hospitals using the same instrument was also reported for comparative purposes to each hospital. The mean value was also reported for each subgrouping under each of the background questions, so that the hospital could see the varying answers from people at different levels, in different areas, and so on, thus pointing out areas in need of help. What follows here is a summary of the major findings for this group of health care facilities.

Overall Evaluation

Table 19-1 shows the answers to five questions dealing with summary judgments about the overall usefulness of MBO:

- Almost four-fifths (79%) have an overall favorable attitude (Q 49).
- Even more, 88 percent, reported MBO effective in helping them as a manager (Q 50).
- Eight-three percent say they are committed to MBO.
- An MBO coordinator was found helpful by two-thirds, with almost one-fourth neutral on this question.
- A total of 89 percent were in favor of continued use of MBO.

Table 19-1 Overall Evaluation

Q 49	What is your overall attitude towards MBO as we are using it here?	
	1. Very favorable	26%
	2. Favorable	53
	3. Undecided or neutral	18
	4. Unfavorable	3
	5. Very unfavorable	0
Q 50	How effective do you feel MBO has been in helping you do your job as a manager?	
	1. Very effective	26
	2. Somewhat effective	62
	3. Neutral	8
	4. Somewhat harmful/ineffective	4
	5. Very harmful/ineffective	0
Q 51	Rate the degree to which you are personally committed to MBO.	
	1. Very committed	39
	2. Somewhat committed	44
	3. Neutral	10
	4. Somewhat opposed	6
	5. Very opposed	1
Q 52	How helpful has it been to have someone officially delegated as MBO coordinator?	
	1. Very helpful	23
	2. Somewhat helpful	43
	3. Neutral	23
	4. Unhelpful	9
	5. Very unhelpful	2
Q 53	What is your recommendation about continuing to work with MBO?	
	1. Strongly in favor	62
	2. Somewhat in favor	27
	3. Neutral	3
	4. Somewhat opposed	6
	5. Very opposed	2

Only two editorial comments might be helpful here. The 24 hospitals had experience with MBO anywhere from 1 year to 3 years. There was a decided tendency for the percentage who voted to continue to use MBO to drop off a little in the institutions with longer experience. In almost every case those negative votes came from individuals who had not been formally trained in MBO, even though the organization had more formal experience with the system. The lesson seems to be that care must be taken to bring newcomers among the management ranks to a satisfactory understanding of the system by carefully providing MBO training for them.

The second comment deals with the lower percentage of those finding an MBO coordinator helpful. The high neutral opinion expressed on this question was from three of the institutions in which a large number of the respondents reported they did not know who the person was. Where the identity was known and where the individual was functioning, there was a high positive response. The lesson seems to be that coordinators must take care to make themselves known. Might one conclude that it doesn't seem to make any difference whether there is a coordinator or not, since all these hospitals still had a high overall satisfaction rate? The answer is that the coordinator is still needed; evidence of this is that other items on the survey reflected less satisfaction in institutions in which the coordinator was not found to be as helpful.

Acceptance, Real Achievement, and Utilization

In this section, seven often mentioned advantages of MBO were cited, and nine frequently heard complaints about MBO were put to the test. Again, five-part multiple choice questions were used.

With regard to the advantages, the hospitals had the greatest success in increasing awareness of the hospital's overall objectives (82% agreed), coordinating work toward the hospital's overall objectives (80% agreed), and enhancing mutual agreement on what is expected between superior and subordinate (79% agreed).

Influencing employees to be humanistic or people-oriented was the lowest scoring in this section, which was very interesting, because very often the charge is made that *all* MBO does is this very thing.

With regard to the common complaints about MBO, the managers disagreed that there was lack of support from top management (74%), lack of any change in behavior due to MBO (75%), and lack of opportunity to update objectives (73%), showing that these are not valid complaints if care is taken to avoid these mistakes in implementation, even though people often "scare" us with such warnings. Other answers indicated that:

- MBO does *not* commit one to a set of inflexible objectives.
- MBO does *not* require too many meetings.
- MBO does *not* tend to be one-way communications.
- MBO *does* fit in well with other planning cycles.
- MBO *is* used by those who should use it.
- MBO is *not* just a fad soon to be forgotten.

Motivation

Concentrating on the self-actualizing aspects of a person's need for motivation, the satisfaction level of the managers using MBO was checked six times. In all of the hospitals, a large majority felt:

- Their work enhanced their self-esteem.
- Their position in the hospital was important.
- They accomplished worthwhile things in their job.
- They had the opportunity for independent thought and action in carrying out their duties.

Slightly fewer than one-half reported that they felt secure in their position and that they had opportunity for self-development.

Three editorial comments are in order. The relatively lower number feeling secure in their position seems to be a common finding after implementation of a system of management that attempts to identify "dead wood." Insecurities tend to surface because inadequacies cannot be hidden when there is an objectives program. You should always expect some turn-over to follow implementation of MBO.

Our second comment concerns opportunity for self-development. Despite the emphasis on personal development objectives and the strong recommendation to make this a part of the MBO program, some organizations skip over that, with the result that managers remember they were promised something they did not get, and this causes dissatisfaction.

Third, it should be pointed out that in three-fourths of the hospitals in this study, the item dealing with opportunity for independent thought and action in carrying out one's duties received the strongest response not only in this set of questions, but in the entire survey. This would seem to underscore the point that MBO need not undermine an individual's freedom for self-expression, as often claimed by the MBO adversaries.

Communications with Superiors

Because one of the major needs addressed by MBO is the common managerial need to bring about and maintain a meeting of the minds between levels of managers, no fewer than 16 items inquired into communications with one's superior.

The ranking of degrees of satisfaction on all these items was never the same in any two hospitals. In most cases, however, there was great satisfaction with the ability to be open and candid during performance review, with genuine interest in one's development, with getting help when problems arise.

There was a second group of items with somewhat less general satisfaction, but still with a high degree of success. These dealt with a clear understanding of how the superior felt about one's performance, with the amount of time spent discussing plans and performance, and with getting feedback on how well one was doing on an ongoing basis. Apparently superiors still need to provide more information to their people about their performance, and this means taking the time to do so—throughout the year and during the performance reviews.

The lowest items of satisfaction, showing a high degree of neutral responses, were those dealing with doing a better job anticipating events, and the superiors emphasizing that managers should manage and not be "doers." Since these get at the very heart of MBO as an anticipatory system of being results-oriented, these are areas needing constant attention.

Objectives Formulation

Writing meaningful and measurable objectives is a planning skill that usually comes with experience. There are certain things we intend and certain others we would like to avoid as we formulate objectives. This section examined a total of five positive items, which might be called desirable, and six negative items, which can be considered undesirable.

In these hospitals, there was a very strong degree of satisfaction with all five desirable aspects of writing objectives:

1. Objectives tended to support the hospital's.
2. Objectives reflected their most important duties.
3. Adequate help was received in writing objectives.
4. Objectives were updated regularly.
5. Objectives were kept handy so they could be looked at from time to time.

Among the undesirable items, three were being avoided:

1. Creativity was *not* being stifled by the objective-writing process.
2. Writing objectives was *not* too much paper work.
3. Objectives *did* contain enough about action plans to help achieve them.

On the other hand, three items in this set received answers generally in the neutral to somewhat dissatisfied area. These dealt with:

1. the ability to measure some result areas
2. the ability to capture routine duties in objectives
3. having enough good data to keep track of some things

To editorialize again, these are the most common areas of difficulty *and are to be expected.* It has been said over and over that it takes three to five years of practical experience for people to feel really comfortable about measuring all their responsibility areas. Part of the reason for this is to be found in these three difficult areas: some will lack good data; some will neglect important areas on their first list or two of objectives; some will need time to figure out significant ways to measure. The following reminders are offered as ways to keep plugging away at these sore spots:

- Work unit measures of productivity could be established in each department with the help of management engineering-type procedures.
- Current statistical reports, activity forecasts, volume measures, and the like should be reviewed for those items of information that are meaningful and can be worked into objectives. If such information is not meaningful enough for objectives, maybe it ought not to be kept any longer, and other information should be substituted in its place.
- Staff positions should seek objectives of a problem-solving and innovative nature, being sure to measure results in terms of anticipated improvements, often as shared by those who are the "clients." The hospitalwide QA program should be a help in pointing out "problem-oriented" objectives for all departments.
- Standards of performance, sometimes stated in a "checklist of conditions desired" form, should be set up for those areas that are more service oriented than production oriented.

SUMMARY

MBO is a tool for managers to use in carrying out their responsibilities. They are the best ones to indicate whether this tool is effective or not. Standard survey techniques can be used to afford them an opportunity to tell administration and the board whether MBO is working.

NOTES

1. For example, Henry L. Tosi in *California Business Review* (Fall 1973).
2. Arthur X. Deegan, "MBO: Does It Work In Hospitals?" *Michigan Hospitals*, Aug. 1981, pp. 16–19.

Bibliography

Abney, Bonnie Maclean. *Blueprint for MBO*. Belmont: Fearon Pitman Publishing, 1979.

American Hospital Association. *Environmental Analysis of the Hospital Industry, 1979*. Chicago, 1979.

Ansoff, H.I. "Company Objectives: Blueprint or Blue Sky?" *Management Review*, Sept. 1962, p. 41 ff.

Barrett, F.D. "The MBO Time Trip." *The Canadian Business Quarterly*, Autumn 1972, p. 42 ff.

Beck, Arthur C., and Hillman, Ellis D. *A Practical Approach to Organization Development thru MBO*. Reading, MA: Addison-Wesley, 1972.

Berne, Eric. *Games People Play*. New York: Ballantine Books, 1973.

Blake, Robert, and Mouton Jane. *The Managerial Grid*. Houston: Gulf Publishing Co., 1964.

Brown, Montague. "The Administrator as Master Strategist." Annual Convocation of American Academy of Medical Administrators, Las Vegas, 1981.

Cardiff, Gary D. "MBO: It Will Work in a Hospital Setting." *Hospital Administration in Canada*, Nov. 1970, p. 23 ff.

Chaite, Richard. "Mission Madness Strikes our Colleges." *The Chronical of Higher Education*, July 16, 1979.

Cotton, Donald B. *Company Wide Planning: Concept and Process*. New York: Macmillan Co., 1970.

Deegan, Arthur X. II. "MBO: Organized Common Sense." *Illinois Libraries*, June 1978, p. 518 ff.

———. *Coaching*. Reading, MA: Addison-Wesley, 1979.

———. "Results Oriented Ambulatory Care Management." *Journal of Ambulatory Care Management*, Feb. 1981, p. 1 ff.

———, and Fritz Roger. *Practical MBO*. Chicago: Deltak Corp., 1976.

———, and O'Donovan, Thomas R. "How Much Authority Should the Administrator Delegate?" *The Modern Hospital*, Oct. 1964, p. 94 ff.

Drucker, Peter F. *The Practice of Management*. New York: Harper & Row, 1954.

———. *The Effective Executive*. New York: Harper & Row, 1967.

———. *Management*. New York: Harper & Row, 1974.

———. "The Dynamics of Health Care Administration." *Federation of American Hospitals Review*, Feb. 1978, p. 14 ff.

Dyck, Merla H. et al. "Goal Setting in Hospital Departments." *Health Care Management Review*, Summer 1981.

Granger, Charles H. "The Hierarchy of Objectives." *Harvard Business Review*, May–June 1964, p. 63 ff.

Greiner, Larry. "What Managers Think of Participative Leadership." *Harvard Business Review*, Mar.–Apr. 1973.

Herzberg, Frederick. "One More Time: How Do You Motivate Employees?" *Harvard Business Review*, Jan.–Feb. 1968.

Howell, R.A. "MBO: A Three Stage System." *Business Horizons*, Feb. 1970, p. 41 ff.

Hughes, Charles L. *Goal Setting: Key to Individual and Organizational Effectiveness*. New York: American Management Association, 1965.

Humble, John W. *Management by Objectives in Action*. London: McGraw-Hill Co., 1970.

Ivancevich, John M. "The Theory and Practice of MBO." *Michigan Business Review*, Mar. 1969, p. 13 ff.

Johnson, Richard L. "The 1980s: The Rise of HMOs and Marketplace Competition." *Hospital Progress*, June 1979, p. e8 ff.

Kahn, Herman, and Briggs, B. Bruce. *Things to Come*. New York: The Macmillan Co., 1972.

Kepner, Charles H., and Tregoe, Benjamin B. *The Rational Manager*. New York: McGraw-Hill Co., 1965.

Kindall, Alva F. "The MBO Approach to Performance Appraisal." *Personnel Administration: Principles and Cases*, 3rd ed. Homewood: Irwin, 1969.

Kuntz, Esther. "Public Law 96-79 Changes Certificate of Need Processes." *Modern Healthcare*, Nov. 1979, p. 50 ff.

Lasagna, John B. "Make Your MBO Pragmatic." *Harvard Business Review*, Nov.–Dec. 1971.

LaViolette, Suzanne. "New JCAH Standard Should Spur Cooperation in Quality Assurance." *Modern Healthcare*, Aug. 1979, p. 34 ff.

Leila, Sr. Mary et al. "Planning: A Full Time Responsibility." *Hospital Progress*, Sept. 1976, p. 94 ff.

Levinson, Harry. "Management by Whose Objectives?," *Harvard Business Review*, July–Aug. 1970, p. 125 ff.

Likert, Rensis. *New Patterns of Management*. New York: McGraw-Hill, 1961.

Mackenzie, R. Alec, and Varney, Glenn H. "The Missing Link in MBO." *Univ. of Western Ontario Business Quarterly*, Autumn 1973.

Mayo, Elton. *Human Problems of an Industrial Civilization*. New York: Macmillan Co., 1933.

McConkey, Dale D. *How to Manage by Results*. New York: American Management Association, 1965.

———. "The Results Approach to Evaluating Managerial Performance." *Advanced Management Journal*, Oct 1967, p. 16 ff.

———. "MBO Works for Managers Who Understand, Apply System." *Hospital Progress*, Sept. 1979, p. 66 ff.

McGregor, Douglas M. "An Uneasy Look at Performance Appraisal." *Harvard Business Review*, May–June 1957, p. 89 ff.

———. *The Human Side of Enterprise.* New York: McGraw-Hill, 1960.

Meyer, Herbert H. et al. "Split Roles in Performance Appraisal." *Harvard Business Review,* Jan.–Feb. 1965, p. 123 ff.

Morrissey, George. *Management by Objectives and Results.* Reading, MA: Addison-Wesley, 1970.

Myers, M. Scott. *Every Employee a Manager: More Meaningful Work Through Job Enrichment.* New York: McGraw-Hill, 1970.

National Laboratory for Higher Education. *MBO Training.* England: David Carpenter Classified Media Ltd, 1971.

Nierenberg, Gerald I. *The Art of Negotiating.* New York: Hawthorn, 1968.

Odiorne, George S. *MBO: A System of Managerial Leadership.* New York: Pitman Publishing Co., 1965.

———. *Management Decisions by Objectives.* New York: Prentice-Hall, 1969.

———. *Training by Objectives.* New York: Macmillan, 1970.

———. *MBO II.* Belmont: Fearon Pitman Pub., 1979.

O'Donovan, Thomas R. "Management by Objectives." *Hospital Topics,* February 1971, pp. 34–37.

O'Donovan, Thomas R., and O'Donovan, Patrick G. "Emergi-centers: The Next Wave," *Health Services Manager,* January 1982.

Osborne, Alex F. *Applied Imagination.* New York: Charles Scribners, 1953.

Perlin, Martin S. "Current Practices in Long Range Planning." *Hospitals,* Sept. 1, 1972, p. 62 ff.

Peter, Lawrence. *The Peter Principle.* New York: William Morrow Co., 1969.

Peters, Joseph P. *A Guide to Strategic Planning for Hospitals.* Chicago: American Hospital Association, 1979.

Pierce, J., and Charles F. "HSA, Hospital Planning: Arena of Conflict Offers Room for Cooperation." *Hospitals,* Mar. 16, 1980, p. 63 ff.

Raia, Anthony P. "Goal Setting and Self-Control." *Journal of Management Studies,* Feb. 1965, p. 34.

———. "A Second Look at Management Goals and Controls." *California Management Review,* Summer 1966, p. 49 ff.

Rakich, J. S., Longest, B. B. Jr., and O'Donovan, Thomas R. *Managing Health Care Organizations.* Philadelphia: W. B. Saunders Co., 1977.

Reddin, W. J. *Establish Your Management Objectives.* New York: McGraw-Hill, 1971.

Ross, David E. "Planning for Survival in Small and Rural Hospitals." *Hospitals,* June 16, 1980, p. 65 ff.

Schleh, Edward C. *Management by Results.* New York: McGraw-Hill, 1961.

Skampa, Jack A. "MBO: A Systematic Way to Manage Change." *Hospitals,* Sept. 16, 1969, p. 49 ff.

Sloan, Stanley, and Schrieber, David E. "What We Need to Know About MBO." *Personnel Journal,* Mar. 1970, p. 206 ff.

Stuehler, George Jr. "A Model for Planning in Health Institutions." *Hospital and Health Services Administration,* Summer 1978, p. 6 ff.

Taylor, Frederick W. *Scientific Management.* New York: Harper & Row, 1947.

Toffler, Alvin. *The Third Wave.* New York: William Morrow, 1980.

Tosi, Henry L. et al. "Managerial Reaction to MBO." *Academy of Management Journal*, Dec. 1968, p. 415 ff.

———. "Some Factors Affecting the Success of MBO." *Journal of Management Studies*, May 1970, p. 209 ff.

———. "Setting Goals in Management by Objectives." *California Management Review*, Summer 1970, p. 70 ff.

Townsend, Robert. *Up the Organization*. New York: Knopf Pub. Co., 1970.

Warner, Robert L. "What and Who of a Quality Assurance Program." Unpublished workshop handout, 1979.

Webber, James B., and Dula, Martha A. "Effective Planning Committees for Hospitals." *Harvard Business Review*, May–June 1974, p. 51 ff.

Winkstrom, Walter S. *Managing By and With Objectives*. Chicago: National Industrial Conference Board, 1968.

Wrapp, H. Edward. "Manage by Objectives or Wheel and Deal?" *Steel*, May 1967, p. 46 ff.

Index

A

Accountability, 35, 36, 317
ACORN, 242
Activities, 10-12, 15
Ambulatory care center, 116
Ambulatory surgery, 80, 81, 103, 104
American Hospital Association, 83, 96
Amniocentesis, 106
Appraisal. *See* Evaluation
Autocratic management, 31-33, 34, 182

B

Base level, 277
Beliefs, statement of, 90
Biofeedback, 106
Biomedical engineering, 106
Blake, Robert, 4
Blue Cross, 98
Board of Directors, 41, 77, 85, 93
Budgeting, 71
Budgets, 155
Bureau of Census, 101

C

California Hospital Association, 79
Career planning, 111
Certificate of need, 74-75, 81
Chaite, Richard, 94
Chief executive officer, 6, 39, 40, 41, 43, 52, 53, 57, 58, 61, 71, 73, 85, 103, 137, 146-147, 260, 297, 309
Cloning, 106
Communications, 21, 64
Comprehensive Health Planning Council of Southeastern Michigan, (CHPC-SEM), 81
Comprehensive strategic planning, 69, 71-72
Controlling, 19, 39
Cost containment, 73-74
Cost reimbursement, 73-74
Credo, 45, 48-49
Cryogenics, 106
Culpability, 35
Cyborgs, 106

D

Decision package, 276-286
Demographics, 100-101, 112
Department heads, 56-57
Department of Health & Human Services, 81
Developmental management, 32-33
Directing, 18, 39
Drucker, Peter, 52, 72, 182, 184, 314

E

Efficiency, 109
Emergency department, 103
Energy, 77
Environmental assessment, 96-97
Evaluation, 156-159
Exception principle. *See* Managing by exception
Expected average, 204, 282
External forces, 73-83

F

Feedback, 72
Fertility rates, 102
Finance, 108
Financial analysis, 102
Follow up, 295-296, 306
Function, 169, 190

G

Ginsberg, Eli, 76
Goals, 15
Gottlieb, Symond, 83
Government, 113
Group training, 59

H

Health maintenance organizations, 98
Health Planning and Resources Development Amendments of 1979, 75
Health services inventory, 101
Health status, 112
Health systems agencies, 74, 76, 79-83, 103
Health systems plans, 79
Hertzberg, Fredericke, 4
Hospital based physicians, 85
Hospital costs, 69
Hospital family, 69-70, 84
Hospital objectives. *See* Objectives
Human resources department, 122

I

Ideals, statement of, 90
Image, 111
Incremental budgeting, 275
Individual goals
  basic assumptions, 1-19
  evaluation, 156
  key results areas, 153
  performance budget, 155
Innovative objectives
  abandonment, 234
  definition, 229
  examples, 235-238
  format, 231-234
Inputs, 9, 11, 14

J

Job description, 62
Job related goals, 182
Johnson, Richard L., 75
Joint Commission on Accreditation of Hospitals, 52, 72, 84, 108, 251-252

K

Kahn, Alfred, 76
Key results areas, 52, 53, 55, 153, 164-175, 184, 185, 193-194, 202, 217
KISS principle (Keep It Short and Simple), 177

L

Likert, Rensis, 4
Line departments, 190
Linking pin organization, 151-152

Long-range planning. *See* Planning

M

Management by Objectives
advantages, 4, 20-25
communication, 6
conceptual framework, 5
definition, 3, 9, 16, 19, 150
disadvantages, 23-24
evaluation, 63-64
feedback, 10
implementation, strategies of, 309-321
objectives, 17
objective setting, 6
practical problems, 4
resolving tension, 6
resources, 14
results oriented management, 9
value added, 10, 12
Management information systems, 60-62, 291
Manager, 7
Managerial grid, 4
Managing by exception, 199-200, 291
Maximum probable, 204, 282
McGregor, Douglas, 4
Medical records, 119
Medical staff, 43, 71, 72, 77, 84, 93, 99-100, 102, 112
Medicare, 71, 98
Minimum acceptable, 204, 282
Mission, 45
statement of, 89-91, 116-122 (samples)
Monthly reports, 291
Moran, David W., 76
Motivating, 18, 22, 39, 64, 93, 327
Multi-hospital systems, 73

N

National Association of Quality Assurance Professionals, 254
National Health Planning and Resources Development Act of 1974 (P.L. 93-641), 74, 75, 83
Needs analysis, 69, 89-114, 96, 102-104
Negotiation, 6
Nuclear medicine, 119
Nursing services department, 117

O

OAK, 242
Objectives
annual, 51, 54, 55, 137-139
definition, 138, 155
local, 80
long-range, 49-50
medium-range, 49, 51
national, 79
short-term individual, 153
state, 79
Outputs, 10, 12, 13-14

P

Participative management, 4, 5, 27, 35, 36, 57, 58
Pastoral care, 119
Patient care division, 120
Performance budget, 155
Personal development goals
commitment from organization, 246
development activities, 245-246
evaluation of achievements, 247
format, 241
success indicators, 243
Personal development needs, 306
Peter, Lawrence, 7
Peter, Principle, 7
Pharmacy, 121
Philosophy, statement of, 46, 91
Planning, 17, 21, 39, 49, 64, 70, 84-85, 123-124
data, 124-133

long-range, 69
operational, 137
strategic, 71, 72, 74, 137
Prioritizing, 146-147
Problem solving objectives
desired performance, 218
identification of problems, 216-217
present performance, 217
sample problems, 224-227
scope of causes, 218
solution development, 221
solution evaluation, 222-224
Psychiatric nursing, 121
Psychosurgery, 106
Public relations, 109-110
Purchasing department, 117
Purpose, statement of, 44, 45, 47, 90

Q

Quality assurance
comparison with MBO, 253-254
implementation, 258-262
Quality control, 108

R

Reimbursement, 73, 74
Results oriented performance review, 299-300
Role, statement of, 90, 92
Routine objectives
critical analysis exercise, 210
desired results, 203
new boss exercise, 205
present level, 201
success indicators, 195-197

S

Self appraisal, 304
Self profile, 28
Service area population, 97, 112
Shared responsibilities, 173
State health plan, 79-80
Statewide Health Coordinating Council, 79
Success indicators
common, 200
cost, 198
exception, 199
number of, 198
quality, 196
quantity, 195
time, 198

T

Targets of opportunity, 294
Technology, 77
Training
department heads, 56-59
supervisors, 59
top management, 41-43
Trend analysis, 104-114

U

Utilization review, 118
Utilization trends, 98

V

Values, statement of, 90
Vitality, 111
Volume of business, 107
Volunteer services, 118

W

Ward, Paul, 79
World War II, 79

Z

Zero based budgeting, 275, 279

About the Authors

DR. ARTHUR DEEGAN is president of Art Deegan and Associates of Clearwater, Florida. He has had more than 18 years of experience designing and conducting management development programs for business firms, government agencies, health care institutions, colleges and universities, and service organizations.

Prior to starting his own consulting firm, he was an associate professor of business administration at the University of Michigan. Since then he has established a national reputation as a consultant in the planning-evaluating process. Dr. Deegan has helped over one hundred different hospitals, both not–for-profit as well as for-profit, to implement MBO.

He has written numerous articles in professional management and trade publications and has authored five books used as the text for intensive workshops or for self-study on MBO and coaching subordinates, including one entitled *MBO for Hospitals*.

Dr. Deegan holds the distinction of receiving a Ford Foundation Fellowship in economics and business administration and a Standard Oil of Indiana Fellowship in industrial relations. His work experience includes ten years as a manager in fund-raising, foreign trade, and hospital administration. He speaks regularly at university-sponsored or company in-house seminars coast to coast.

THOMAS R. O'DONOVAN is the president of the American Academy of Medical Administrators in Southfield, Michigan. From 1964 to 1979 he was the administrator and chief operating officer of Mount Carmel Mercy Hospital and Medical Center in Detroit, Michigan.

Dr. O'Donovan received his bachelor's and master's degrees in management from the University of Detroit, and a Ph.D. in management from Michigan State University, where he majored in administrative management, corporation finance, marketing, and economics. From 1956 to 1964 he taught at Michigan State University, University of Detroit, and the University of Southern California.

The author of over 90 scientific papers, articles, and reports that have been published in various health care and other journals, he has also been a program director of over 30 conferences and has delivered a speech or made a scientific presentation at over 100 educational conferences and programs. He is a Fellow in the American Academy of Medical Administrators, in the College of Hospital Administrators, and in the Royal Society of Health. In 1971 Dr. O'Donovan was recipient of the William Newcomer Award as "The Medical Administrator of the Year" presented by the American Academy of Medical Administrators. He has been a member of the editorial board of the journal *Hospital and Health Services Administration,* published by the ACHA, for over seven years.